Frontiers in Biology and Medicine

The Human Body: Origins and Complexity

The Bacteria within Us: Human Microbiome and our Health

The Human Genome and Individualized Medicine

Curing Genetic Disease with Gene Therapy

Regenerating our Organs: Regenerative Medicine

The Power of Stem Cells

Thomas C. Spelsberg, Ph.D.

Illustrators: Kenneth D. Peters
Thomas C. Spelsberg, Ph.D.

The sculpture shown on the front cover page is titled "Man and Freedom" by the Croatian sculptor, "Ivan Mestrovic." The photograph is courtesy of the Mayo Foundation for Medical Education and Research; used with permission.

Thomas C. Spelsberg, Ph.D., has been on staff at the Mayo Clinic for over 40 years. He is a Named Professor of Biochemistry and Molecular Biology, and a Distinguished Investigator at the Mayo Clinic. He was born and raised in Clarksburg, West Virginia, and received his BA (biology and chemistry) and Ph.D. (genetics and biochemistry) from West Virginia University. Dr. Spelsberg then became a fellow, and subsequently a faculty member, in the Department of Biochemistry at the University of Texas M.D. Anderson Hospital and Tumor Institute at Houston, TX (now known as the University of Texas M.D. Anderson Cancer Center). In 1970 he joined the faculty of reproductive biology at Vanderbilt University Medical Center, and while there, was awarded the National Genetics Foundation Scholarship. He then joined the Mayo Clinic in 1973 as an Associate Professor in the Department of Biochemistry and Molecular Biology; Professor in 1975.

Dr. Spelsberg has served as section head and then chair for the Department of Biochemistry and Molecular Biology (1988-1995). From 1984 to 1994, he served as the director and principal investigator of the NIH-funded Mayo Clinic Center for Reproductive Biology. Dr. Spelsberg holds the George M. Eisenberg Professorship and was named the first Distinguished Investigator at the Mayo Clinic. He has also received several teaching awards from the students in the Mayo Graduate and Medical Schools. He has mentored 68 pre- and post-doctoral fellows. In 1988 he was elected secretary of the Officers and Councilors by the Mayo Clinic Staff and then elected in 1995 as the first Ph.D., President of the Mayo Clinic Staff. From 1999 to 2005, Doctor Spelsberg served as Mayo Clinic's Director of Medical Genomics Education Program.

Over his career, he has served on National Institutes of Health (NIH) review boards, various national committees, foundations, institutions, and advisory boards, and numerous editorial boards for scientific journals. He was elected to the Council of the American Society for Bone and Mineral Research and to the West Virginia University Academy of Distinguished Alumni. Dr. Spelsberg was also appointed to the National Advisory Board for the West Virginia University Health Sciences Center.

He is internationally recognized for his research on the mechanisms of action of steroid hormones, hormone antagonists, growth factors, and transcription factors in human breast cancer and skeletal disease. He currently holds 12 U.S. patents and has been awarded numerous grants over the past 40 years from the NIH, and private foundations.

He has authored over 360 publications, and has presented over 50 symposia and plenary lectures. Over the past 15 years, his fellows have received 40 national and international awards for their research. He is a member and past president of the Board of Directors for the George M. Eisenberg Foundation for Charities of Chicago.

Preface

Audience interest spanning 30 years from lectures at the Mayo Clinic and Mayo's sponsored meetings inspired Dr. Spelsberg to write this book for physicians, allied health professionals, teachers, and the public (young and old) who have an interest in the sciences. These lectures on Frontiers in Biology and Medicine, include the following topics: "Origins and the Micro-universe of the Human Body," "The Human Microbiome," "The Human Genome," "Gene Therapy," "Individualized Medicine," and "Regenerative Medicine." These lectures were presented to the Mayo Clinic staff, alumni, fellows, allied health professionals, and medical/graduate students. This book presents facts about the origins of the atoms and molecules that make up our bodies, the micro-universe of the human body and the cells which compose it, the bacteria which live on and inside us and affect our health, the human genome and what makes us individuals. This is followed by some important breakthroughs which have occurred in biology and medicine in areas of gene therapy, individualized medicine, and tissue regeneration.

"It is difficult for students to learn when they are hungry and unloved or live in homes with violence, abuse, and no direction."

The Author

Acknowledgements

The author would like to thank the following individuals for the preparation of this book: My family (Liza, Sarah, Thomas, and Nancy), my many Mayo colleagues and research collaborators who encouraged me to convert these lectures to a book. My wife, Liza, and daughter, Nancy, were instrumental in editing, formatting, and publishing this book; my son, Thomas, who designed and formatted the front cover; Ken Peters, who designed many of the excellent illustrations and tables. Thank you, Jackie House, for your excellent clerical support throughout this process and Eric Wieben, Ph.D., Director of Medical Genome Facility, Mayo Clinic and Graduate School of Medicine, for serving as an excellent resource for the various scientific facts and processes. Thank you to all the proof readers for your excellent revisions and advice: Ursula Iwaniec, Ph.D. and Russ Turner, Ph.D., research scientists at the Oregon State University; Sarah Spelsberg, physician's assistant in orthopedic surgery, Mayo Clinic Florida; Nalini Rajamannan, MD, cardiologist, Chicago, IL, and Anne Gingery, Ph.D., assistant professor, Mayo College of Medicine.

This book is dedicated to my loving family, Liza, Sarah, Thomas, Nancy, daughter-in-law Katie, and grandchildren, Tommy, Ruby, and Walter, and to the Mayo Clinic staff all of whom have given me excitement and great joy over the years.

Contents

Chapter 1

Prologue

The chapters of this book present biological and medical topics in descriptive terms with many tables and figures. The information presented is taken from the author's lectures and a variety of books, journal articles, and reputable web sites, some of which are listed at the end of the book. The various tables and figures were taken from power point lectures presented by the author, or are originals designed specifically for this book. These models, tables, and diagrams are intended to replace lengthy text with the concept that "a picture is worth a thousand words." This book is designed to avoid overwhelming you with intricate descriptions. Therefore, the various concepts are simplified in order to provide an easier understanding of the exciting world of biology and medicine.

The book is organized into 5 sections, ranging from molecules to the human body. These are:

I)   The Human Body

II) The Human Microbiome and our Health

III) The Human Genome and Individualized Medicine

IV) Curing Genetic Disease by Gene Therapy

V)   Regenerating Our Organs: Regenerative Medicine

Chapters 2 and 3, "Cosmic Origins of Humans" and "The Beginning of Life" describe where all things on Earth originated, and the possible origins of life. This is followed by Chapter 4, "The Micro-universe of the Human Body and the Cells that Compose It" which describes the complexity of the human body and the human cell. This complexity is compared to various structures in the celestial cosmos, and helps explain why medical advancements are so difficult to achieve. Chapter 5, "The Microbial World: The Vast Numbers and Their Symbiotic Social Life," and Chapter 6, "The Human Microbiome and Our Health: The Massive Bacterial World within Us," describes the universality and multitude of symbiotic bacteria which live within us and are needed for our well-being. Subsequent chapters (7–12) describe, in broad terms, the fundamental approaches, ongoing progress, and future possibilities of important areas of medical research: "The Human Genome," "How Genes and Epigenetics Create the Human Individual," "The Future Roles of Individualized (Personalized) Medicine," "Curing Genetic Diseases with Gene Therapy," "The Power and Universality of the Human Stem Cells," and finally, "Current Achievements in Regenerative Medicine." Each chapter begins with definitions of important terms within that chapter. These are also compiled at the end of the book. General references for each chapter are listed at the end of the book under "References for Further Reading."

This book is meant to excite, educate, and inspire science oriented young and lay audiences, as well as medical professionals and educators. Readers will learn about the amazing and wondrous world of the human body, the genes that control it, and exciting advances in biology and medicine. Each chapter is presented in concise, easy-to-read sections. The author hopes this book will educate and inspire the public to support education and research, and will encourage young adults to consider careers in the exciting worlds of medicine, medical research, and teaching. Above all, the author hopes that readers will enjoy the amazing facts, philosophies, and messages about life, our microbial friends, our bodies, and promises from new discoveries in medicine. By the way, this book was fun to do.

Section I

The Human Body: Origins and Complexity

Chapter 2

Cosmic Origins of Humans

Definitions

<u>atoms</u>: smallest particle of chemical elements that contains the chemical properties of that element; comprised of a nucleus of protons and neutrons surrounded by orbiting electrons.

<u>compound</u>: substance formed by the chemical bonding of 2 or more different elements/atoms into molecules.

<u>cosmos (universe)</u>: The universe, i.e., everything in the universe, including stars, planets, nebulae, galaxies, etc.

<u>cyanobacteria (blue green algae)</u>: a phylum consisting of 2 groups of photosynthetic bacteria which use the sun to produce its food and energy, and use water to produce oxygen.

<u>elements</u>: basic form of substances found on Earth that cannot be broken down.

<u>galaxy</u>: a huge cluster of stars (islands) numbering in the billions in the cosmos.

<u>molecules</u>: the smallest units of a compound that maintains the chemical properties that compound; a group of atoms forming a stable unit, i.e., a compound that can be divided.

<u>nova</u>: a relatively small star that explodes within milliseconds, creating heavier atomic elements, and over a period of weeks or months becoming thousands of times brighter.

<u>nucleofusion/nucleosynthesis</u>: The combining of lighter-smaller atoms of elements into heavier, larger atoms to create new elements under extremes of temperatures and pressures – occurs in the centers of stars during their life and during their exploding deaths.

periodic table: a table listing the elements according to increasing atomic number, which is based on the numbers of protons in their nuclei – the arrangement correlates with their chemical and physical properties.

supernova: The explosion of a large star – (eight or more times the mass of our sun), that fuses under extreme conditions, the nuclei of lighter elements to create the heaviest of elements, i.e., iron and all those heavier than iron. This occurs in milliseconds to seconds. Temperatures in the billions of °F and pressures 100 billion times that of Earth's gravity create these heavier elements. Supernovae are extremely bright, brighter even than the whole galaxy comprised of 100-200 billion stars. The brightness lasts a few weeks.

universe: see cosmos above.

A.   Introduction

We often take our Earth (land and water), the sun, stars, and living creatures, including ourselves, for granted – for just being there and for functioning properly. However, all of us must have wondered at one time or another about the origins of the sun, stars, and the earth, including the elements such as gold, diamonds, and iron. Being an amateur astronomer, it has always been of interest to the author to understand the origins of the molecules and elements (atoms) which make up earth, our cells, our bodies, and life in general. This chapter will give the readers a perspective on the origins and ages of the chemical elements on Earth. Scientists do not know the answers to all these questions, but a surprising amount is known. The first section of this chapter begins with the origin of the universe (cosmos). This section is followed by the creation of the elements that compose all living organisms and everything on Earth. Table 2.1 is designed to help the reader learn about the various numerical connotations, including the powers of 10, the English nomenclature, and the International standard nomenclature, in dealing with the vast numbers mentioned in this book. These numerical connotations are used in Chapters 2–7 to describe the complexities of the human cell, human body, and the microbial world, including the microbes within us. Further reading on the topics in this book can be found at the end of this book under "References for Further Reading" for Chapter 2.

B.   A Global Picture of the Cosmos

Let us begin with a global picture of the cosmos and Earth. Today we look up to the heavens and see approximately 2000 stars with just our eyes on a good night. However, we can see hundreds of billions of stars with large telescopes. We know that our solar system is in the outer regions of the Milky Way Galaxy, pinwheel of 200 billion ($2x10^{11}$) stars, many of which are believed to have planets. Our galaxy is part of a "local group" of a dozen or so galaxies which is part of a still larger group of galaxies, the Virgo Supercluster, and so on. There is a minimum of 100 to 200 billion galaxies in the visible universe (cosmos), each galaxy having 100 to 300 billion stars. The term "visible universe" is used because it is speculated that a lot more of our universe (estimated to be 6-7 times more) is not visible, as it is too far away and its light has not reached us yet. All of these galaxies are structured in walls or filaments (of galaxies) surrounding voids of empty space. These empty voids between the walls of galaxies, and the walls themselves, are now believed to also contain the mysterious, invisible, "Dark Matter" which represents 96% of the total matter in the universe. This dark matter is now thought to help create the structures of galaxies and walls of galaxies and voids using its gravitational force. Scientists now believe that the stars are also held together in galaxies (islands of stars in a sea of space) not only by their own mutual gravities, but by the gravity of this mysterious, invisible, dark matter.

The total visible universe contains anywhere from 10^{22} to 10^{23} stars (10 x billion x trillion stars) (table 2.1). Scientists estimate there to be an even greater number of planets, possibly 10 times the number of stars. This would calculate to about a trillion (10^{12}) planets in our galaxy alone. Scientists have recently estimated that our Milky Way has approximately 8.8 billion Earth-like planets that have a climate similar to Earth's climate. Even if only 1 out of 10,000 planets has life on it, there would be 100 million (10^8) planets with life in the Milky Way galaxy, or one billion x one billion (i.e., one quintillion) planets with life among the hundreds of billions of galaxies in our visible universe.

Table 2.1

Numerical values, symbols, terms, and prefixes				
Number	Exponent	Standard International	English	Approximate diameter (in meters)
0.000,000,000,000,000,000,000,001	10^{-24}	Yocto	one septillionth	Neutrino
0.000,000,000,000,000,000,001	10^{-21}	zepto	one sextillionth	
0.000,000,000,000,000,001	10^{-18}	atto	one quintillionth	Quark
0.000,000,000,000,001	10^{-15}	femto	one quandrillionth	atomic nucleus
0.000,000,000,001	10^{-12}	pico	one trillionth	helium atom
0.000,000,001	10^{-9}	nano	one billionth	glucose molecule
0.000,001	10^{-6}	micro	one millionth	Bacteria human cell
0.001	10^{-3}	milli	one thousandth	
0.01	10^{-2}	centi	one hundredth	
0.1	10^{-1}	deci	one tenth	
1.0	10^{0}	- -	one	Human
10	10^{1}	deka	ten	
100	10^{2}	hecto	hundred	football field
1,000	10^{3}	kilo	thousand	
1,000,000	10^{6}	mega	million	Earth
1,000,000,000	10^{9}	giga	billion	sun (star)
1,000,000,000,000	10^{12}	tera	trillion	largest star
1,000,000,000,000,000	10^{15}	peta	quadrillion	Oort cloud
1,000,000,000,000,000,000	10^{18}	exa	quintillion	Nebulae
1,000,000,000,000,000,000,000	10^{21}	zetta	sextillion	Galaxy
1,000,000,000,000,000,000,000,000	10^{24}	yotta	septillion	hubble deep field
1,000,000,000,000,000,000,000,000,000	10^{27}	--	octillion	Universe

How did our universe begin? Computer analysis of distances and velocities of galaxies support the big bang theory as the beginning of our universe, the origin of which occurred approximately 13.7 billion years ago as a subatomic point. The universe first underwent a super expansion called "inflation." It is also known that galaxies (or group of galaxies) are now speeding away from each other as a result of the "Big Bang" with the addition of another mysterious force, called "dark energy," which is speculated to be accelerating this expansion in the last billion years or so. Scientists are now attempting to understand the big bang theory and even trying to theorize what existed "before" the big bang and what will occur at the end of our expanding universe. What is known is that, within seconds after the big bang, which began with temperatures of 100s of billions °F, protons and neutrons began to form and received their mass from the Higgs Boson particles.

By 380,000 years post the big bang, the extreme temperatures lowered to a level (less than 10–20 billion °F) whereby whole atoms consisting of protons, neutrons, and electrons, were able to come together to form small, simple, light weight elements, such as hydrogen, deuterium (an isotope or subclass of hydrogen), helium, and lithium. By 200–300 million years after the big bang (approximately 13.5 billion years ago) the first stars and galaxies began to form. These were comprised of only the original light elements, such as hydrogen, deuterium, helium, and lithium. Gaseous planets (like Jupiter and Saturn) also probably formed to create solar systems along with the stars. There were no rocky planets, as the heavier elements composing them did not exist. It is estimated that the peak of star formation occurred 3 billion (3×10^9) years after the big bang, i.e., or about 10 billion years ago.

C.   The Origins of the Elements (The Building Blocks of all Visible Matter)

There are 92 naturally occurring elements (atoms) on Earth, beginning with the lightest, hydrogen, and ending with the heaviest, uranium. Scientists believe these also occur throughout the universe. The 92 elements are organized in the periodic chart (hydrogen to uranium) according to their number of protons (atomic number) (see table 2.2). The periodic chart represents the elements composing the known (visible) matter on Earth. These elements are also detected in the cosmos (e.g., in stars, nebulae, planets, and moons). These known elements, in the form of atoms, are the fundamental building blocks of all things, living and non-living. As depicted in figure 2.1, it was approximately 13 billion years ago when the 89 heavier elements, i.e., elements heavier than hydrogen, helium, and lithium, began to be created in the centers of stars and during the death of stars by a process called nucleosynthesis. This process involves the fusion (combining) of the atomic nuclei of the lighter elements which requires a lot of energy.

Nucleosynthesis occurs in the center of stars at temperatures in the hundreds of millions to a few billions of degrees Fahrenheit. The fusion is assisted with pressures estimated to be as high as 300,000 times Earth's gravity. As outlined in figure 2.1, the 23 elements heavier than lithium, e.g., carbon, neon, oxygen, silicon, calcium, up to iron, are now known to be synthesized deep inside stars through nucleosynthesis. These stars end up having an onion like structure with bands of the newly created heavier elements located closer to the center of the stars. The lighter of these elements (carbon, neon, oxygen) are synthesized in small to average size stars. The heavier of these elements (calcium, iron) are synthesized in larger stars. In contrast, the 66 heaviest elements, – additional iron and all heavier elements up to uranium, – are now known to be created in a few milliseconds, during the implosion/explosion of stars (called novae and supernovae) at the end of a star's life. The creation of the heaviest elements requires even higher temperatures (approximately 5 to 9 billion °F) and pressures [approximately millions to billions Earth's atmosphere (1 atmosphere=14.7 pounds per in^2)], which cause the fusion of heavy elements to create even heavier elements. Further details of the creation of the elements can be found in figure 2.1.

For the past approximately 13 billion years, all of these heavier elements from star explosions end up in the leftover remnants (clouds) originating from these explosions. These clouds are called nebulae. Thus, the 23 heavier elements up to iron, created in the hot centers of pre-existing stars, as well as the 66 heavier ones (up to uranium), created during their exploding star deaths, were then used to form new stars and planets. As time progressed, the new suns and planets were created not only of hydrogen, helium, and lithium, but also with ever increasing amounts of the heavier elements. The heavier elements began to appear in new stars and created the solid "rocky" planets, moons, asteroids, and comets.

By 9 billion years after the big bang (4.5 billion years ago), our own sun and solar system began to form from the gas nebulae which were generated from the novae and supernovae remnants (nebulae) of the pre-existing first/second/third generation stars and their solar systems. Our solar system nebula contained all the elements (heavy and light) we find today on Earth. All the nebulae and stars throughout the Milky Way galaxy and other galaxies appear to contain the same elements (at varied ratios) as found on Earth and on our sun. Interestingly, as discussed at the end of this chapter, many of these elements, generated in our

Table 2.2

PERIODIC TABLE OF THE ELEMENTS

Table 2.2: The Periodic Table of Elements. The elements are arranged in rows called periods. The elements are also arranged in rows in order of their atomic number, i.e., the number of protons in the nucleus. The elements in the vertical columns are called groups or families whose members have the same properties.
Taken from: J.I. Lunine, 1999, "Earth" Cambridge University Press, NY, NY.

Figure 2.1

Synthesis of All the Elements Found on Earth by Fusion of Smaller Atomic Nuclei into Larger Atomic Nuclei in Stars

(Before the Earth and Solar System were born)

Age (Years Ago)	Cosmic Events	Temperatures at Nucleosynthesis (Fusion of Atoms)	Elements Created
~ 13.7 Billion (10^9)	Big Bang	~ 10^{32} °F (Trillions of Trillions °F)	Hydrogen, Helium, and Lithium
~ 13 Billion	Star Cores Small Stars (x 0.1 sun)	~ 20×10^6 °F (20 Million °F)	Hydrogen Helium
	Middle Stars (x 1–4 suns)	~ 200×10^6 °F (200 Million °F)	Lithium Carbon
	Large Stars (x 4–50 suns)	~ $1–3 \times 10^9$ °F (1–3 Billion °F)	Nitrogen Oxygen Sodium
		~ $3–5 \times 10^9$ °F (3–5 Billion °F)	Magnesium Calcium Iron
	Death of Stars (Novae, Supernovae)	$5–9 \times 10^9$ °F (5–9 Billion °F)	Iron Silver Iodine Platinum Gold / Silver
5.0 Billion			Uranium
4.5 Billion	**Birth of Solar System and Earth**		**Utilizing all of the above**

(© Thomas C. Spelsberg and Kenneth D. Peters 2012)

cosmos, are the same elements that make up living things. This fact was the basis of the statement by Carl Sagan, "We're made of star stuff."

It should be noted that there are also an additional 11 or so laboratory-produced elements that have been created by man, e.g., plutonium, americium, curium, and californium. It is important to remember that, as discussed earlier, 96% of the universe's total matter with gravity remains of an unknown structure and is known as "dark matter." This dark matter is invisible (i.e., does not interact with light), and only its gravitational effects can be measured. Scientists have yet to identify what it is.

D.   The General Structure of the Elemental Atoms and their Compounds (Minerals)

Atoms are the fundamental unit of elements that consist of a nucleus (containing neutrons and protons) surrounded by a "halo" of electrons. The increasingly heavier elements have increasing numbers of neutrons, protons, and electrons. Each species of atom, representing each element, has its own specific composition of protons, neutrons, electrons, and chemical properties. It is interesting to note that 99.999% of an atom represents "empty space," as the atomic nucleus is so small relative to the electron halo revolving around it. For example, picture a sphere with a diameter the size of a football field. Add a few marbles in the center of the sphere (50 yard line) to represent the atomic nucleus, and add electrons flowing around the surface at the end zones. The rest of the space in the sphere is the empty space. Thus, the solid items around us which we use, handle, and interact with, are in reality 99.999% empty space. Many of the elements combine chemically with each other via sharing, receiving, or donating electrons with each other, to create larger molecules known as minerals, such as salts, limestone, and gypsum. These minerals (also called compounds) represent the primary form in which all of the elements on Earth are found. It will be exciting to understand the composition and structure of the mysterious dark matter of our cosmos.

E.   Ages of the Elements

As deduced from previous discussion, the lighter hydrogen, helium, and some lithium elements are as old as the universe itself, or approximately 13.7 billion years old. The elements on Earth, that are heavier than lithium, range in age from 6 to 12 billion years old, and were created long before the earth was formed (only 4.5 billion years ago). As described above, during the first 9 billion year period, the nebulae from exploded stars were used to rebuild new stars and solar systems, including our solar system. Thus, the carbon in the foods we eat, the gold, silver, and platinum we admire, the oxygen and nitrogen we breathe, the water and ethanol (hydrogen and oxygen) we drink, and the copper and iron with which we build things, contain the atoms of elements which are 6–12 billion years old. These ages should give us an appreciation of the elements that compose our everyday foods, utensils, and us. All things, including living organisms, are truly made from "star stuff."

F.   Origins and Ages of the Sun, Earth, and Solar System

The solar system, including the sun and Earth, were formed approximately 4.5 billion (4.5×10^9) years ago from a nebulae created by the deaths of pre-existing stars. These stars had previously synthesized all of the 89 elements listed in the periodic chart (table 2.2), and which are naturally found on Earth, that are heavier than hydrogen, helium, and lithium. Thus, Earth was built about 4.5 billion years ago from a nebula of stardust that was generated with the material from the death and debris of small to large stars that existed 5–12 billion years ago. This dust cloud then condensed to planet Earth by gravity. Our moon was created 4.35 billion years ago, shortly after the earth was formed, from the debris of a planetary impact of early Earth.

G.   Origins and Ages of Earth's Atmosphere, Water, and Land

    (1)   The Atmosphere

Recent isotope analyses indicate that much of the atmosphere and ocean water originated from the nebula, which condensed to create Earth and our solar system. A lesser amount of minerals (and water) came from comet and asteroid impacts. The land masses of Earth were created approximately 3–4.5 billion years ago by the huge uplifting of Earth's mantle and extreme volcanism. About 4.0 billion years ago, during the Hadean eon, Earth's original atmosphere, contained little oxygen, i.e., it was anaerobic. Most of the oxygen was in the form of iron oxides and water. Thus, life is speculated to have begun approximately 3.8–4.3 billion years ago with extreme living bacteria (extremophiles) in an atmosphere which was very toxic by today's standards. Obviously, the planet's atmosphere we breathe today is nothing like the first half of Earth's existence. This low oxygen atmosphere lasted for 2.5 billion years.

Earth's atmosphere began to change around 2.5 billion years ago at the start of the proteozoic eon, when photosynthesizing bacteria [cyanobacteria or blue green algae, classified as prokaryotes (bacteria)] in the oceans began producing oxygen. Using energy from the sun, large volumes of oxygen were generated from water by the sun's energy (photosynthesis), which evolved in the prokaryote cyanobacteria, and created the oxygen-rich atmosphere we enjoy today. The oxygen levels in the atmosphere peaked at 20-30% oxygen about 500-700 million years ago, which started the Cambrian Era. This high oxygen generated a massive increase in the living species, including multicellular organisms, e.g., insects, plants, and animals, including the dinosaurs. The atoms making up our atmosphere, created 5–12 billion years ago, have been recycling again and again on Earth. It stands to reason that some of the air molecules we breathe today were previously inhaled by ancient organisms (e.g., bacteria, dinosaurs, and mammoths) and early humans (e.g., Julius Caesar, George Washington, Abe Lincoln, and John Kennedy).

(2)   Human Pollutants

As an interesting side note, humans now add significant chemicals to Earth's atmosphere, e.g., 250,000 tons of formaldehyde per year from car exhaust, and wood and coal burning, etc., 375,000 tons of benzene and 2 million tons of ammonia per year both from industrial sources. Further, as of 2010, the burning of fossil fuels generated approximately 25 billion (25×10^9) tons each of carbon dioxide and methane, as well as thousands of tons of sulfur dioxide, nitrogen oxides, thorium, uranium, and other heavy metals. A recent study reported that a typical cubic meter of office and household air also contains, in addition to the above chemicals, several hundred fungal spores, 89 micrograms (μg) of ethanol, 42 μg of acetone, and 16 μg of formaldehyde and acetone. In addition, we breathe 100 million microbes per minute in an average household (discussed in Chapter 5), as well as fragments of cockroaches and dust mites. I'm sure all of this is not refreshing to hear (or breathe).

(3)   Water

Recent analyses of atomic isotopes of hydrogen in the earth's water has led to the conclusion that the majority of the water on Earth was directly introduced as part of the gas nebulae from which the earth originally formed about 4.5 billion years ago. These isotope studies suggest that asteroids and comets delivered only a small amount of water to the earth between 3.5 and 4.0 billion years ago. The original water of the condensing nebulae is speculated to have been vaporized by subsequent asteroid and comet impacts, but remained in the Earth's atmosphere as water vapor. In any case, the water molecules have also been recycled and reused for billions of years in one physical state or another. It is interesting to note that the water we drink could have been used by bacteria and algae billions of years ago, by dinosaurs 200 million years ago, by giant sloths and saber-toothed tigers 25 million years ago, by Moses and Christ 2000-3000 years ago, Thomas Jefferson 250 years ago, and Einstein 100 years ago.

(4)   Land – Earth's Crust and Us: We are made of Clay

Land is comprised of minerals whose elemental atoms were also created 6–12 billion years ago in previously existing stars, as described earlier. Thus, the components of the land originated from the solar nebulae, generated by past exploding stars. Table 2.2 shows the elemental composition of humans (and all animals for that matter) compared to that of the Earth's crust. All of the elements in the Earth's crust and atmosphere are found in life forms on Earth at one level or another, including humans. In fact, carbon, oxygen, hydrogen, and nitrogen compose 96% of the matter of living organisms. These elements also represent four out of the five most abundant elements on the earth's crust. Only the chemically inactive helium is missing in life forms. Furthermore, 8 out of the 12 most abundant elements in the Earth's crust (clay) are also among the most abundant elements making up the human body (see table 2.3). About 20 additional elements are found in minute levels in living organisms as well as in the crust.

Table 2.3

Elements Found in the Human Body and Earth's Crust
(in order of abundances)

Top Elements in Humans (Percent of Body Mass)	Top Elements in Earth's Crust and Atmosphere
1. 65% Oxygen	1. Oxygen
2. 18% Carbon	2. Silicon
3. 10% Hydrogen	3. Aluminum
4. 3.0% Nitrogen	4. Iron
5. 1.4% Calcium	5. Calcium
6. 1.1% Phosphorus	6. Sodium
7. 0.2% Sulfur	7. Potassium
8. 0.2% Potassium	8. Magnesium
9. 0.14% Sodium	9. Titanium
10. 0.12% Chlorine	10. Hydrogen
11. 0.1% Magnesium	11. Nitrogen
	12. Carbon

Taken from: J. Emsley, Nature's Building Blocks, 2001,
Oxford University Press

Figure 2.2

Outline of Life's Building Materials

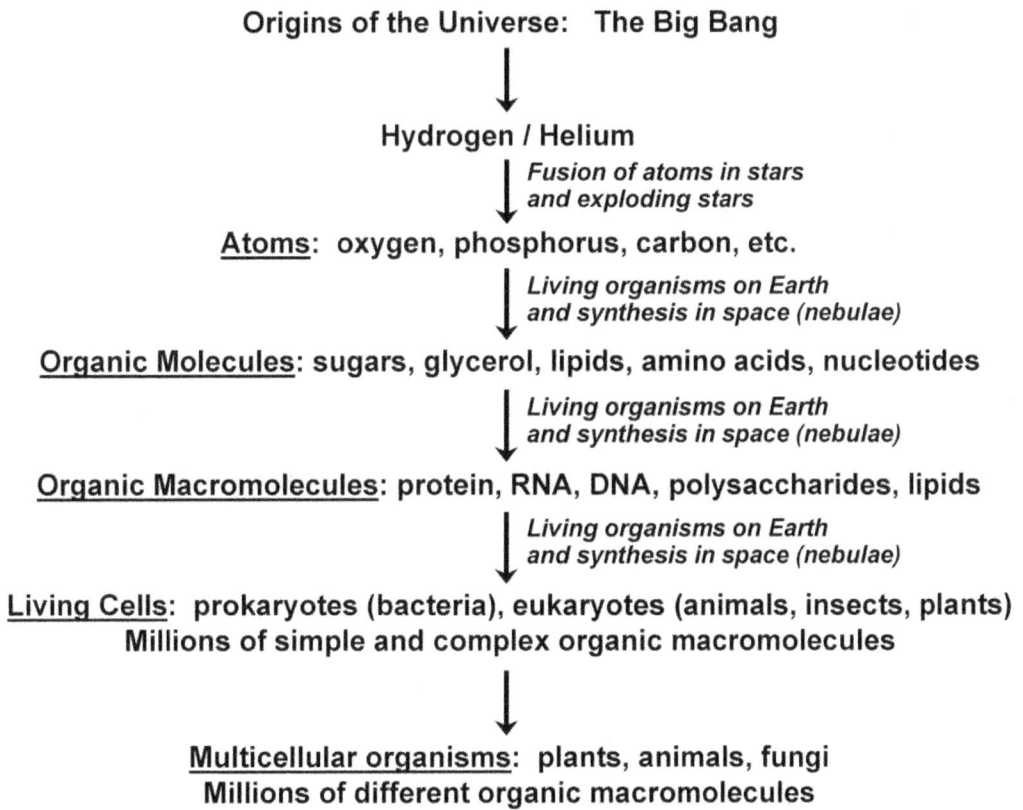

Origins of the Universe: The Big Bang

↓

Hydrogen / Helium

↓ *Fusion of atoms in stars and exploding stars*

Atoms: oxygen, phosphorus, carbon, etc.

↓ *Living organisms on Earth and synthesis in space (nebulae)*

Organic Molecules: sugars, glycerol, lipids, amino acids, nucleotides

↓ *Living organisms on Earth and synthesis in space (nebulae)*

Organic Macromolecules: protein, RNA, DNA, polysaccharides, lipids

↓ *Living organisms on Earth and synthesis in space (nebulae)*

Living Cells: prokaryotes (bacteria), eukaryotes (animals, insects, plants)
Millions of simple and complex organic macromolecules

↓

Multicellular organisms: plants, animals, fungi
Millions of different organic macromolecules

(© Thomas C. Spelsberg and Kenneth D. Peters 2012)

It is interesting to note that science agrees, in this instance, with the Bible in that mankind and all living things are made of clay. Only aluminum, silicon, magnesium, and titanium, which are only minimal levels in our bodies, are more abundant elements in Earth's crust. Life obviously did not need large quantities of these. If life began on another planet/moon, maybe our human composition more accurately reflects the composition of that planet. Considering our cosmic origins, it is likely that the various elements in each of our bodies came from different stars. To add to the old philosophical statement, all life goes through the cycle of "ashes to ashes and dust to dust," we now might add the scientific version, "elements to elements."

H.   Origins of the Inorganic Minerals and Organic Molecules

As mentioned earlier, most elements combine together to create minerals (salts, acids, gypsum, etc.) which are the common form of elements on Earth. These are inorganic molecules. As described earlier, minerals are also called "compounds" (meaning to put together as in the union of separate elements). Minerals are created by the natural, spontaneous, chemical binding of two or more different elements. Minerals are the natural form of most elements on Earth and are represented by salts, acids, gypsum, sand, natural gas, water, and more. While the elements on Earth are classified as inorganic, the organic molecules (arising from living organisms) represent more complex (larger) molecules primarily comprised of carbon, along with oxygen, hydrogen, phosphorus, and nitrogen. Even though a few small organic molecules/compounds can occur naturally (chemically synthesized) in the environment and are found in the cosmos (e.g., nebulae and comets), they have been termed organic since living organisms produce most of the organic compounds found on Earth, especially the complex compounds. Figure 2.2 lists the origins and increasingly complex organic compounds found in living creatures on Earth. As depicted in figure 2.2, these organic molecules can be small (e.g., amino acids, sugars, and lipids) or large [e.g., proteins (comprised of many amino acids), polysaccharides (comprised of many sugars), complex lipids (comprised of many lipids) or even a combination of these (such as lipopolysaccharides and lipoproteins)].

I.   The Dollar Value of the Human Body

Did you ever wonder what the human body is worth in terms of its inorganic (elemental/mineral) and organic molecular composition? It has been estimated that the human body, reduced to its basic minerals (elements), is worth about $2.00 on today's market. However, according to Kowles, 2010, ("The Wonders of Genetics"), the value of the average human body in terms of large organic/biologically active molecules (i.e., proteins that include hormones, enzymes, growth factors and cytokines, which are synthesized by the cells of our bodies), is about $6–8 million or more. We can relax, as our lives are still safe with these valuable items, since the isolation of these molecules would cost more than they are worth. Further, the similar functioning molecules can be found in all mammals (dogs, cows, pigs, horses, etc.) and some can be synthesized in the laboratory by bacteria or animal cells. Thus, we are safe from personal destruction by financial zealots.

J.   Origins of Our Gold, Silver, Diamonds, and Gems

It is interesting to ponder the history of the heavy elements (platinum, gold, and diamonds) in our jewelry, that we so admire and for which we pay handsomely. Most diamonds (crystals of carbon) in one's jewelry were created deep in Earth's lower mantle (terrestrial), but a few were brought in by asteroids (extraterrestrial) or created by comet/asteroid impacts. Earth's upper core and lower mantel domains are estimated to have pressures ranging from 0.3 to 3 million (3×10^6) atmospheres (45 million pounds per square inch), and temperatures from 3,000 to 8,000°F, which are more than enough to create diamonds out of carbon and other gem stones. These minerals were brought to the surface via volcanism, since the heavier elements settled to the Earth's core when the young Earth was a molten mass. Most diamonds are tens of millions to a few billions years old, while the gold and platinum in which they are set are even older, i.e., created 6–12 billion years ago in dying stars. In any event, when you admire jewelry, you should also admire and ponder the ancient/primordial history of the material composing it.

K.   Matter is Never Lost, but Recycled

As discussed above, nothing (or very little) on Earth and in the universe is lost or used up. It is always recycled. All the elements on Earth, such as hydrogen, oxygen, gold, and iron, including the elements in the air we breathe, the water we drink, and the food we eat, are constantly recycled to be used again. Even matter comprising past living organisms has been recycled into new living organisms again and again. Each of our breaths contains approximately 10^{22} gaseous molecules (10 x billion x 1 trillion molecules) of the elements and compounds (e.g., carbon dioxide, hydrogen, oxygen, and water). Each breath surely contains the molecules breathed by past living organisms on Earth tens of millions to billions of years ago. Thus, as mentioned above, we breathe the same air molecules that could have been used/breathed from 200 million to 4 billion years ago by bacteria, algae, animals (dinosaurs, giant sloths, mastodons), or more recently by humans. The same recycling occurs with water, food, and all minerals. To be accurate, we should mention that there are gains in material on Earth from comet/meteorite impacts and "cosmic dust" settling on Earth, to the amount of 100 tons per day. However, there are also slight losses of material from Earth, caused by the solar wind stripping away some of our upper atmosphere.

L.   Conclusions

Our Earth and all living creatures are made of elements and resulting minerals (compounds) which were created in the cosmos. Many of these elements and minerals are billions of years old, and have been used by other living creatures over the past 4 billion years on Earth. Nothing is lost on Earth, but is recycled over and over. There is truly an atomic connection between humans and our universe. Humans and all living things have cosmic origins and are comprised of star stuff.

Chapter 3

The Mysterious Beginnings of Life

Definitions

algae: a class of protista, mostly single cell eukaryotes that live in water, most using photosynthesis as plants but others using chemical energy as animals.

Archaea: One of two subkingdoms (phyla) of bacteria. The other is eubacteria. Many of these live in extreme environments, and are called extremophiles. This subkingdom is thought to represent the first forms of life on Earth.

DNA (deoxyribonucleic acids): genetic material in the chromosomes of the cell nucleus containing hereditary genes comprised of deoxyribose sugars and the nitrogen containing base units.

eukaryotes/eukarya (a superkingdom): a kingdom of organisms comprised of complex cells which contain a nucleus and true chromosomes represent plants, animals, insects, fungi, and protista: some scientists classify this category as a superkingdom, the other being prokaryotes.

kingdoms: highest level of taxonomic classification: includes prokaryotes (archaea and bacteria) and eukaryotes (plants, animals, insects, etc.).

kingdom Animalia: represents all animals; also classified as a superkingdom; represents eukaryotes whose cells lack cell walls and undergo embryonic development of egg-blastula-gastrula-adult.

kingdom fungi: acellular eukaryotes that lack chlorophyll and function as parasites or symbionts.

kingdom Monera (prokaryotes): kingdom representing all the prokaryote bacteria, including the two phyla called eubacteria or archaebacteria; some scientists classify this category as a superkingdom.

kingdom Plantae: eukaryote organisms comprised of cellulose wall and chlorophyll; these organisms are autotrophs: organisms that synthesize their needed organic materials from inorganic sources using the sun or geothermal or chemical energy.

kingdom Protista: kingdom comprised of unicellular and multicellular eukaryote algae, protozoa, fungi, plants, and animals.

macromolecules: large, multicomponent organic molecule usually comprised of carbon atoms linked together [e.g., proteins, polysaccharides (sugars) and lipids (fats)].

organic molecules: molecules produced by living organisms that are comprised of carbon, hydrogen, and sometimes oxygen, nitrogen, and phosphorus.

phylums: primary taxon (subgroup) of kingdoms.

prokaryotes (bacteria) (a superkindom): compose the kingdom of Monera, which do not contain a nucleus or true chromosomes; the other superkingdom is eukaryotes.

RNA (ribonucleic acid): single stranded nucleic acid and ribose sugar containing bases; has multiple functions such as gene expression and cellular structures.

species: a taxonomic category consisting of closely related individuals which can interbreed to produce fertile offspring.

A.   <u>Possible Origins of First Life</u>

We are always amazed and perplexed when we ponder how and why life got started. The bottom line is, we do not know. There are many books and articles written about the origins of life, but all of these only represent educated guesses. The topic is interesting to consider, but there is currently no absolute answer. Therefore, all the theories and scientific writings on the subject will not be given much discussion in this book. Admittedly, thinking about life's origins over a glass of wine can put one in a spiritual mood. As discussed in Chapter 2, all living things are comprised of elements and their compounds found in Earth's crust. These life elements include six major elements: carbon, hydrogen, oxygen, sulfur, phosphorous, and nitrogen. These same elements are found in abundance in Earth's crust in the form of minerals (i.e., combinations of atoms of elements).

Although mankind has seemingly figured out the origins of the cosmos, its structure, galaxies, the life and death of stars, as well as the origins of all the elements, we can only guess about the origins of life. How did it start? Did life on Earth actually start on another planet or solar system in the cosmos? Whatever the origins, about 3.8–4.3 billion years ago, shortly after Earth was created, these atoms and minerals somehow combined into macromolecules, some really big, such as DNA, RNA, proteolipids, and polysaccharides, as well as into large structures, such as chromosomes and membranes of cells. These macromolecules were used to create life with the ability to reproduce. How these molecules were able to create self-replicating living organisms (cells) is unknown. Once life was initiated, a selection for survival by the environment followed. Scientists have identified the fossils of bacterial-like organisms that are approximately 3.5 billion years old with chemical evidence of life as old as 4.3 billion years old, at the beginning of the Archean eon.

Interestingly, astronomers have detected many simple organic molecules, i.e., simple building blocks of life, in the gas clouds (nebulae) in space. They have detected sugars, amino acids, small lipids, ethanol, acetylene, formaldehyde, cyanide, methanol, formic acid, and even the nitrogenous "bases" which are the building blocks of our genetic material (DNA). It is speculated that these were created by physical-chemical means and provide scientific support that many organic molecules can be derived by "natural chemical bonding," as demonstrated in the laboratory. In fact, using combinations of elements, – heat, anaerobic (low oxygen) gasses (hydrogen and methane), cyanide, and water, – scientists have been able to create complex organic compounds in the laboratory, such as amino acids (the building blocks of proteins), nitrogenous bases (nucleotides: building blocks for RNA and DNA), and even short strands of RNA and DNA (the genetic material).

One wonders whether some of these organic molecules fell to Earth via comets to help generate life here. One has to also consider that life actually could have begun somewhere else in the cosmos and "fell" to Earth, as proposed by the Greek Philosopher, Anaxagoras, ~2,500 years ago and embellished in modern times by Drs. Fred Hoyle and Francis Crick among others. This process is called "panspermia." Scientists have speculated that life probably began with replicating molecules, the most plausible being RNA as opposed to DNA. RNA can replicate itself, and even carry out chemical (enzymatic) reactions. Other scientists argue that life began with proteins. In any case, only guesses can be used in the creation of life. We also do not know how quickly this occurred, but it is theorized that life started more than once, only to be extinguished and restarted. Some scientists speculate that the creation of life probably involved double-layered lipid membranes somehow creating containers (cells) with enzymatic proteins that could generate energy via sunlight or chemicals (sugars or chemical bonds) and replicate themselves to create the earliest living "organisms." The story has been expanded with the addition of "clay" surfaces or semi-liquid colloidal gels assisting in this organization. Some scientists speculate that life started at specific geological locations such as hot vents deep on the ocean floors, or in frigid ice conditions at Earth's poles where organic molecules were squeezed together in air pockets in ice, forcing cellular organization.

To conclude, we do not know how life got started. Based on the fossil history of life on Earth and the dangerous solar radiation in early times, it is probable that life started in the oceans. As stated earlier, some astronomers think that life could have been delivered to Earth by comets and asteroids in the process called panspermia.

B.   First Life: Bacteria and Not Viruses

Fossil evidence suggests the earliest life forms were bacterial like (prokaryotes). Chemical evidence suggests that they first appeared on Earth at approximately 3.8–4.3 billion years ago, and they ruled Earth alone for another 2 billion years (until 2 billion years ago). There is evidence that the more advanced "eukaryote" cells, which make up humans, plants, animals, etc., and other multicellular organisms, began approximately 1.8–2.0 billion years ago. The first "detectable" (fossil) life has been classified under the "kingdom Monera" representing the Archea and Eubacteria Prokaryote phyla (bacteria) (see figure 3.1). Bacteria are single cell organisms, averaging about one-tenth the size of human eukaryote cells. Bacteria lack nuclei, membrane bound organelles, and a strict compartmentalization of metabolic domains. In the scientific community, these cells are known as prokaryotes (*in front of – or – before – nuclei*) and are much simpler and smaller organisms than the eukaryotes. Details of bacteria, especially as they relate to humans, are discussed further in Chapter 5. Some might argue that viruses which infect bacterial and eukaryote cells are the simplest and thus might be the first life. However, viruses cannot live/reproduce alone as can bacteria and, as parasites of bacteria (called phages), must have appeared after bacteria were thriving and used them to reproduce in order to survive as they do today.

As stated above, we do know from fossil records that life began approximately 3.8–4.3 billion (10^9) years ago, during the Hadean and Archean eons, about one-half billion (500 million) years after Earth was created (i.e., 4.5 billion years ago). Life began without much oxygen; it probably used chemical energy, to create a simple prokaryotes (bacteria) under extreme conditions. Examples of such ancient bacteria today are the extremophiles that are discussed below. As outlined in figure 3.1, the members of this bacteria kingdom (Monera) are divided into distinct domains (phyla) of Archaea (ancient or founding bacteria, including extremophiles), and the Eubacteria, in which well known bacteria, such as E-coli, are classified.

The first bacteria that appeared in the fossil record are the extremophiles that are classified under the Archaea bacteria phylum. These are still a major domain of life on Earth. The bacteria of this class live in the extremes of Earth's environment, miles below the ocean surface in hydrothermal vents, miles beneath the land surface and beneath the ocean bottoms, in dry deserts, in hot geysers, in salt lakes, and in rocks and glaciers. As discussed later in Chapter 5 and outlined in table 5.2, the members of extremophiles are subclassified as thermocidophiles (heat and acid lovers), psychrophiles (cold loving), acidophiles (acid loving), alkaliphiles (alkali loving), methanogens (methane breathers), barophiles (high pressure loving), halophiles (salt loving), xerophiles (dry loving), or anaerobes (oxygen hating). Some barophiles live under high pressures (approximately 10,000 times the surface air pressures) miles below the ocean and land surfaces. Psychrophiles live in subfreezing temperatures in Earth's polar regions. Many of these bacteria do not require oxygen, and thus, are classified as anaerobes. They utilize elements such as iron, hydrogen, hydrogen sulfide, methane, etc., in place of oxygen to generate energy. It is this phylum of Archaea that represent the major organisms which degrades/eats dead organisms. They are the ones generally involved in spoiling foods and creating bad odors as well.

As outlined in figure 3.1, the phylum, Eubacteria (true bacteria), are best represented by cyanobacteria (formerly blue-green algae). It is the cyanobacteria of this group that are also believed to have generated Earth's oxygen via its primitive form of photosynthesis beginning approximately three billion years ago. The mitochondria found in animal cells and the chloroplasts found in plant cells are believed to be derived from this class of bacteria (discussed below). It is not known exactly the total number of species that exist under the kingdom Monera (Prokaryotes) (see Chapter 5).

C.   Eukaryote Cells with Nuclei and Chromosomes Composing the Kingdoms of Protists, Plants, Animals, and Fungi

As indicated in figure 3.1, various members of the bacteria kingdom are

Figure 3.1

Classification of Living Things

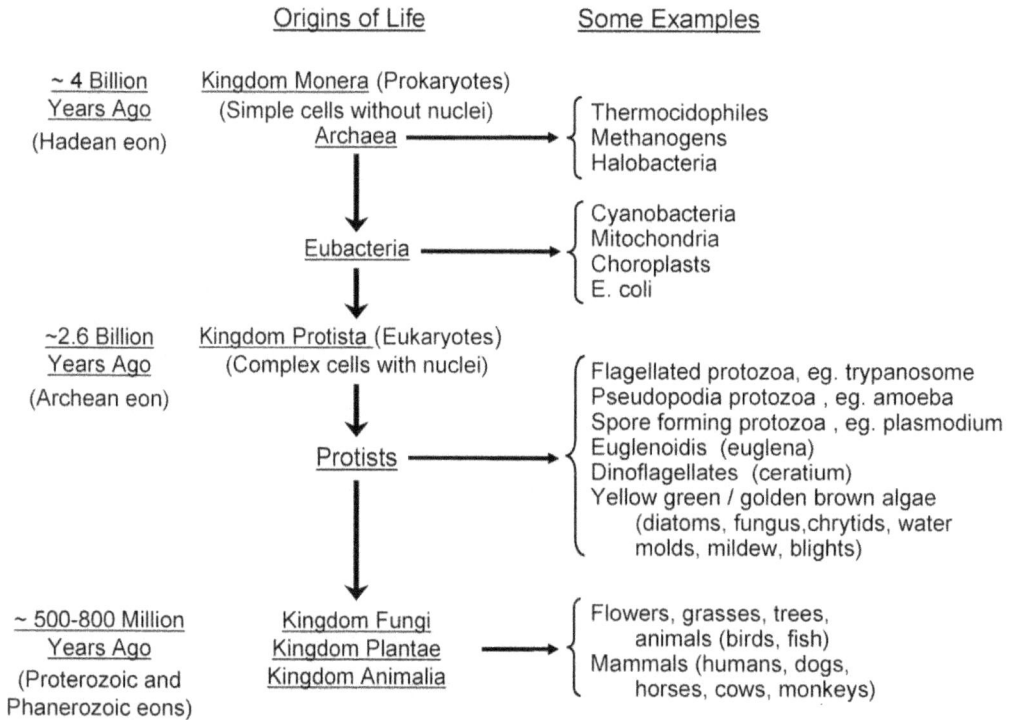

Origins of Life   Some Examples

~ 4 Billion Years Ago
(Hadean eon)

Kingdom Monera (Prokaryotes)
(Simple cells without nuclei)
Archaea ⟶
{ Thermocidophiles
Methanogens
Halobacteria

Eubacteria ⟶
{ Cyanobacteria
Mitochondria
Choroplasts
E. coli

~2.6 Billion Years Ago
(Archean eon)

Kingdom Protista (Eukaryotes)
(Complex cells with nuclei)

Protists ⟶
{ Flagellated protozoa, eg. trypanosome
Pseudopodia protozoa , eg. amoeba
Spore forming protozoa , eg. plasmodium
Euglenoidis (euglena)
Dinoflagellates (ceratium)
Yellow green / golden brown algae
    (diatoms, fungus,chrytids, water
    molds, mildew, blights)

~ 500-800 Million Years Ago
(Proterozoic and Phanerozoic eons)

Kingdom Fungi
Kingdom Plantae
Kingdom Animalia ⟶
{ Flowers, grasses, trees,
    animals (birds, fish)
Mammals (humans, dogs,
    horses, cows, monkeys)

(© Thomas C. Spelsberg, PhD 2012)

believed to have combined by endosymbiosis (joined/living together) to produce the eukaryote cells about 1.8–2.6 billion (approximately 2 thousand million) years ago. Figure 3.2 diagrams the relative sizes of living entities to help you gain a better perspective of the complexity and sizes of these organisms. The organelles inside the cells of the superkingdom, Eukaryotes, called mitochondria and chloroplasts, are now believed to have originated as engulfed bacteria by other bacteria which established a mutually beneficial cohabitating relationship (symbiotic). This is the process that is thought to have created the superkingdom of eukaryotes beginning with the kingdom of Protista (i.e., the simplest organisms comprised of eukaryote cells). These eukaryote cells ultimately served as the beginnings of four kingdoms: 1) Protista (represented by protozoa, algae, molds, and diatoms); 2) Fungi; 3) Plantae; and 4) Animalia (including mammals and primates). The Protista kingdom of eukaryotes consists of many single cell members/species and is estimated to have evolved two billion years ago as one cell (unicellular) organisms. The kingdoms of multicellular organisms, Fungi, Plantae, and Animalia, subsequently evolved in the oceans later, around one billion years ago. A recent genetic analysis estimates that plants and animals separated from common ancestors about one billion years ago.

Gradually, the ozone layer around the Earth developed from the oxygen rich atmosphere, which reduced the harmful solar radiation and allowed the early animals and plants to survive on land. Soon thereafter, at the beginning of the Cambrian era (approximately 500–700 million years ago), multicellular organisms, such as plants and animals, began to thrive in the oceans, lakes, and on land, due to the high oxygen levels in the atmosphere. Interestingly, new studies indicate that bacteria (prokaryotes) played a role in the eukaryote development. Recently, scientists have identified a factor, produced by bacteria, that encourages them to fuse together; this trait could well explain eukaryote cell formation. A study by Nicole King and colleagues at the University of California at Berkley, found that bacteria release substances which encourage both unicellular bacterial and eukaryote cells to colonize into multicellular entities/species (N. King, 2012, Science 33: 510) Further, it has recently been found that when bacteria are eaten by unicellular eukaryote organisms, some of the bacterial genes join with the DNA/chromosomes of these single and multicellular eukaryote organisms in a process called "horizontal gene transfer." This process grants the eukaryote cells with new (bacterial) traits. As stated above, one such trait has been identified as the ability in single cell eukaryotes to form multicellular status as bacteria can do. It is estimated that there are 5–50 million eukaryote species of life on Earth with more recent estimates of 8–20 million.

One recent assessment indicates that approximately 6.5 million species of the phylum, Protista (eukaryotes), reside on land, and 4.2 million in the oceans. Another recent estimate has animals representing 7.8 million species, insects representing 3.7 million species, fungi representing 611,000 species, and plants representing 300,000 species. Interestingly, of these many millions, only a total of about 1.9 million species of all life forms (about 10% of the total) have been classified with names. A 2011–2012 expedition called "Tara Oceans" surveyed the world's oceans, from the surface to one kilometer deep for all living, floating small life forms, viruses, bacteria, plankton, archea, protists, fish larvae, and other small metazoans. They found 1.5 million different taxa (organisms), with most of these never before identified. It should be noted that an estimated 99% of all the species of multicellular eukaryote organisms that have ever lived are now extinct.

Figure 3.2

Relative Sizes of Living Organisms

Plant / Animal Cell:
20×10^{-6} meters
(Diameter)

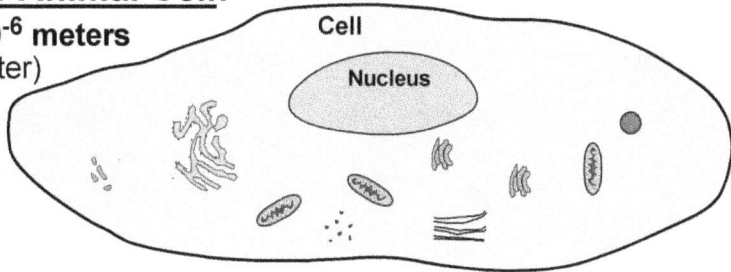

Bacterial Cell:
2×10^{-6} meters
(Diameter)

Virus:
0.08×10^{-6} meters
(Diameter)

(© Thomas C. Spelsberg and Kenneth D. Peters 2011)

The constant creation and extinction of species of life forms is a common pattern of life on Earth.

Chapter 4

The Micro-universe of the Human Body and the Cells that Compose It

Definitions

enzymes: a protein with the power to perform biochemical reactions at a high rate and specificity.

exosomes (extracellular): extracellular nano-vesicle originating from one cell and merging with another. These vesicles transfer lipids, DNA, RNA, and protein (in the form of regulatory RNAs, growth factors, and hormones) from one cell to another and often affect the biology of the neighboring cell.

homo sapiens / sapiens: the modern species of today's humans: classified under the order "primates" and genus "homo."

human cells: basic living unit of human bodies (and all eukaryotes): a eukaryote cell type with protoplasm surrounded by a plasma membrane and containing a nucleus and mitochondria; there are approximately 200 types of human cells in the human body.

lipids: small and large molecules comprised of chains of fatty acids, chains of carbon and oxygen with side groups sometimes attached; used in physical structures, signaling molecules, some enzyme activities, etc.

nucleic acids: see DNA and RNA in Chapter 3.

nucleus: an organelle in a eukaryote cell with 10% of the cell volume containing the cell's chromosomes with DNA (genetic information), as well as the DNA replication and gene expression machinery.

paracrine and cytokine factors (see growth factors): chemical signal molecules which act as cell-to-cell communicators between cells; can be a neurotransmitter or hormone. Involved in regulating cell differentiation and cell metabolism.

proteins: large molecules comprised of linear chains of amino acids. These chains fold to create specific structures, some as components in structures in the cell, some to carry out enzymatic (chemical) reactions.

A.   Introduction

Now that we have discussed the origins of things, including life itself, let's assess what has evolved in terms of our favorite animals, the primate humans (*homo-sapiens sapiens*). We usually take our bodies and their functions for granted until we are sick. This chapter discusses the complexities of the human cell and the human body, as one of the reasons medical research progresses slowly. It also takes a look at the amazing way cells and organs of the human body functions in a cohesive fashion. The individual human cell and the human body will be introduced as complex micro-universes rivaling the complexity of our cosmos (universe). Interesting facts and numbers regarding the composition of the human body are included to give the reader an appreciation of this micro-universe. This vast complexity of the human body should give you an appreciation of the difficulties encountered by the medical research community in elucidating the various causes and treatments of human diseases.

It should be noted that in addition to the molecular complexities of the cell/body composition, there is added complexity due to cell-to-cell communications, cell turnover, cell death, tissue/organ regeneration, and ongoing essential "life" processes in the human body – these processes are only briefly described here. For reference sake, the author and his illustrator have outlined the dimensions of the human body, the organs, the cells and their organelles, and the macromolecules in figure 4.1. This provides a perspective on the various areas and sizes of the entities discussed in this chapter, but they are not drawn to scale, as you would not be able to see anything below the human organs.

B.   The Micro-universe of our Human Body

    (1)   Our Bodies are Astronomically Complex

As outlined in table 4.1, the human body is itself a micro-universe, at least in terms of the number and complexities of its components. Each of our bodies contains approximately 12,000 miles of blood vessels, as well as 10 to 100 billion (10^{10}–10^{11}) neurons, 100 trillion (10^{14}) neuron connections, and an estimated whole body total of 10 trillion (10^{13}) cells. Some people may speculate that large bodies have a lot more cells, but the numbers are roughly the same. Let's consider one organ of the body, the brain, as an example. Again, I imagine some of us may also think that some people have less neurons, but the numbers are roughly the same. It appears that it is the number of connections between individual neurons that makes the difference in intellect. The human brain represents 2% of the body weight, but uses 20% of the total body's energy. It is estimated to have a storage capacity of 1 quintillion (1×10^{18}) bytes of information with 1 quintillion operations per second. There is little wonder that over 250 brain diseases are known and no computer to date can match one average human brain operation.

To give a better appreciation of these values, the author, being an amateur astronomer, has included table 4.2, which compares the numerical composition of components in a human body with those in the cosmos. The number of cells in the whole human body (10 trillion) is 100 times greater than the number of stars in the Milky Way galaxy, while the number of neurons in our brains is about the same as there are stars in the Milky Way galaxy (100 billion). It has been calculated that there is a total of 6 feet of double-stranded DNA (our genetic information found in our chromosomes) in each of the 10 trillion cells of the human body. As listed in table 4.1 and 4.2, if the DNA in all the 10^{13} cells/humans were placed end to end, and multiplying 10^{13} cells/human x 6 feet DNA/cell, one obtains a value of 10 to 12

Figure 4.1

Dimensions and Components of the Human Body

Dimensions

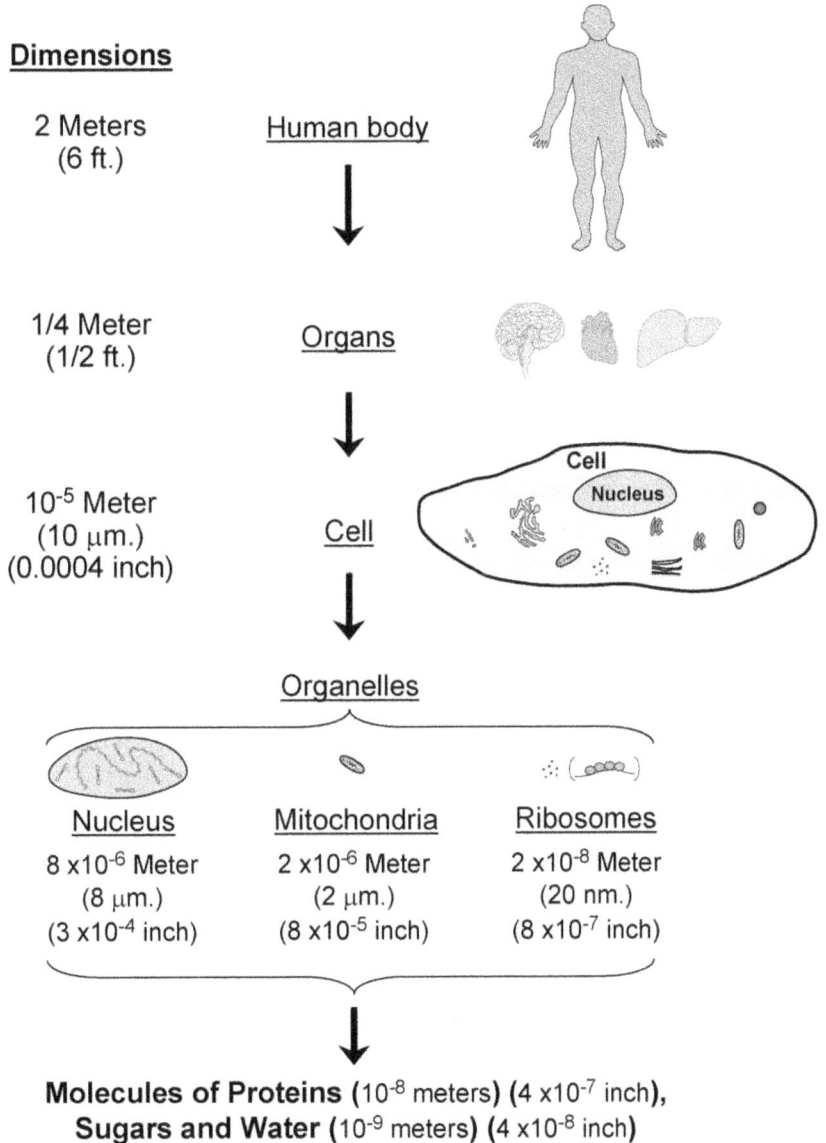

Dimensions		
2 Meters (6 ft.)	Human body	
1/4 Meter (1/2 ft.)	Organs	
10^{-5} Meter (10 μm.) (0.0004 inch)	Cell	

Cell

Nucleus

Organelles

Nucleus	Mitochondria	Ribosomes
8×10^{-6} Meter (8 μm.) (3×10^{-4} inch)	2×10^{-6} Meter (2 μm.) (8×10^{-5} inch)	2×10^{-8} Meter (20 nm.) (8×10^{-7} inch)

Molecules of Proteins (10^{-8} meters) (4×10^{-7} inch)**,
Sugars and Water** (10^{-9} meters) (4×10^{-8} inch)

Table 4.1

Complexity of One Human Body

Entity	Number
Human Body	1
Types of Cells/Body	~200
Cells/Body	~10 Trillion (10^{13})
Blood Vessels	~12,000 Miles
Neurons in one Brain	~10–100 Billion (10^{10}–10^{11})
Neural Connections (Synapses) in one Brain	~100 Trillion (10^{14}) to 1 Quadrillion (10^{15})
Total Nerve Fibers in one Brain	~100,000 Miles
Internal Surface Area of the Lung	~100 Square Yards
Total Membranes in one Human Liver	~6 Football Fields
Total DNA Length/Body	~10 Billion Miles (12×10^9)
Molecules/Cell	~10–100 Trillion (10^{13}–10^{14})
Molecules/Body	~1 Octillion (10^{27})
Cells Created/Destroyed Each Day	~100 Billion (10^{11})

(Thomas C. Spelsberg, 2012)

billion miles of DNA per human body. This length of DNA would stretch from Earth to the moon and return (for a round trip total of 480,000 miles) about 25,000 times, or take 60 round trips from Earth to the sun. How is this possible? It is possible because the DNA strand is so very thin (approximately 1/billionth of a meter in diameter), which makes a typical chromosomal strand of DNA (approximately 3-4 inches long) 40 million times longer than it is wide. For example, if the width of a DNA strand were enlarged to ¼ inch, e.g., the width of a pencil, the length of DNA in each chromosome would be 4000 miles long, a distance greater than that between New York and Los Angeles. Thus, the DNA can be compacted a billion (10^9) fold to reduce the 6 feet of DNA/cell to a small ball less than a micron (1/millionth of a meter), or about 1/3 millionth (3×10^{-7}) of a foot, in diameter. The genetic complexity of our DNA is further discussed in Chapter 7.

(2)   Our Cells are Created and Destroyed by the Billions Each Day

Another amazing fact listed in table 4.1 is that the cells in our body are in constant turnover, being created and destroyed every minute, hour, and day. It is estimated that approximately 10 billion (10^{10}) of our cells are created and destroyed each day, i.e., 400 million each hour. This occurs in our skin, blood, and organs. These 10^{10} cells represent approximately 1/1000 of the total cells in the human body. Besides generating body heat and carrying on life essential cell and organ functions, especially in the brain, cell turnover consumes the major part of our daily nourishment. The greatest number of turnover of our cells occurs in our intestines with the dead and discarded cells eliminated in the feces. A large number of dead cells is also shed from our skin (the largest organ by weight in the body). It is estimated that we shed 1.5 million cells per hour from our skin alone. Every time we take a step or rub our hands, eyes, scalp, etc., hundreds to thousands of cells drop to the ground. This explains why your dog (and other animals) can sense your presence and accurately track your trail/migration. They can do this even on a chronological (time) basis since the more recently dropped cells emit the stronger scent than the older dropped cells. Thus, the movies are accurate, when describing a person crossing a stream or river. The discarded cells would be dispersed quickly in the river, destroying the trail of your cellular odor and the dog's ability to track you.

Many cells are also being destroyed and replaced ("turnover") in all tissue/organs of the body, including bone, muscles, fat, lung, etc., and even in the heart. In old age, the rate of turnover decreases, resulting in an increase in damaged, aged cell population. In some locations more cells are destroyed than created, resulting in a loss of function. As with all mammals, some cells in our bodies are days old, while others are months old, and some (neurons, skeletal osteocytes) are many years old. Our major nerve cells are as old as we are, but all of the cellular components are continually being renewed (replaced). This subject of cell life and regeneration is further discussed later in Chapter 11, "Regenerative Medicine: The Power and Universality of the Human Stem Cell."

C.   The Micro-universe of Human Cells

(1)   Each of our Cells is a Universe in Itself: A Micro-universe

Each of the cells in our bodies is as complex as our bodies, but at smaller dimensions. Table 4.3 lists some of the estimated values highlighting the complexity of each one of the trillions of cells in our bodies. Amazingly, each cell of the 10 trillion cells in our bodies represents a micro-universe in itself.

Table 4.2

The Micro-universe of the Human Body (Numbers compared to our world and the cosmos)			
Equivalent values			Approximate equivalent values
Exponential Number	Numerical No.	English Term	
10^0	1.0		Human body
10^1	10	Ten	DNA/cell in feet
10^2	100	Hundred	Cell types/human
10^3	1,000	Thousand	
10^4	10,000		
10^5	100,000		
10^6	1,000,000	Million	
10^7	10,000,000		
10^8	100,000,000		Earth to sun in miles
10^9	1,000,000,000	Billion	
10^{10}	10,000,000,000	10 Billion	Humans on the Earth; DNA/human body in miles
10^{11}	100,000,000,000	100 Billion	Neurons (cells) in brain; Stars in Milky Way Galaxy; Daily cell turnover/body; Humans that have ever lived
10^{12}	1,000,000,000,000	Trillion	Galaxies in universe
10^{13}	10,000,000,000,000	10 Trillion	Cells / human body
10^{14}	100,000,000,000,000	100 Trillion	Molecules / human cell; Bacteria in/on human body; Neuron connections in brain
10^{15}	1,000,000,000,000,000	Quadrillion	
10^{16}	10,000,000,000,000,000		
10^{17}	100,000,000,000,000,000		
10^{18}	1,000,000,000,000,000,000	Quintillion	Storage capacity of brain; Operations/second in brain
10^{21}	1,000,000,000,000,000,000,000	Sextillion	Total stars in visible universe
10^{24}	1,000,000,000,000,000,000,000,000	Septillion	
10^{27}	1,000,000,000,000,000,000,000,000,000	Octillion	Total molecules in human body
10^{31}	10,000,000,000,000,000,000,000,000,000,000		Number of bacteria on the Earth

(Thomas C. Spelsberg, 2012)

The average human cell weighs only 1 billionth of a gram (2 trillionths of a pound) and on the average has been measured at 10-50µm (~1/1000 of an inch) in diameter. Some cells can be as large as 100µm (100 microns or 1/100th of an inch). Neurons, of course, can even be larger. As also shown in table 4.3, a cell weighing 1 billionth of a gram and measuring 1/1000 of an inch in diameter has been calculated to contain 75-80% water, 10% protein, 6% RNA, 2% fat, and 1–2% metabolites. Obviously, since cells make up our bodies, these molecular values are similar to those of the whole human body.

Most impressive are the enormous molecular populations associated with these percentages. For example, it has been estimated that each cell contains up to 100 trillion molecules (10^{14}). Most of these molecules are water, but still there are an estimated approximately 60 billion protein molecules, one billion RNA molecules, and trillions of fat, sugar, amino acids, and more. As discerned from Tables 4.2 and 4.3, there are 1000 times as many molecules in each of our cells (100 trillion) than there are stars in the Milky Way (100–200 billion). As shown in table 4.2, the total number of molecules in each of our bodies (water, lipid, RNA, and protein molecules) is 1 x octillion (approximately 10^{27}) which is 100,000 times the total number of stars in the whole visible universe, estimated to be approximately 2 x 10^{22} stars. (or 20 x billion x trillion). The latter value is obtained by the fact that there are 200 billion (2×10^{11}) Milky Way-like galaxies, each with approximately 100 billion (10^{11}) stars. Thus, 2x 10^{11} galaxies x 10^{11} stars = 2 x 10^{22} stars. As a multicellular organism, human bodies are truly complex, as are our individual cells.

Table 4.3

Micro-universe of the Human Cell

I. Physical Dimensions*

Weight of average cell	1 billionth ($\sim10^{-9}$) of a gram ($\sim$1 trillionth of a lb)
Diameter of average cell	1 thousandth ($\sim10^{-3}$) of an inch
Surface of average cell	10 millionth ($\sim10^{-7}$) of a square inch (6.45×10^{-7} cm^2)
Volume of average cell	1 billionth ($\sim10^{-9}$) of a cubic inch ($\sim52 \times 10^{-9}$ cm^3)

II. Molecular Composition of a Typical Cell*

By Mass	By Molecules
75% - 80% water	100 trillion ($\sim1 \times 10^{14}$)
10% protein	60 billion ($\sim60 \times 10^{9}$)
6% RNA	1 billion ($\sim1 \times 10^{9}$)
2% fat	2 trillion ($\sim2 \times 10^{12}$)
1.5% metabolites (sugar, etc)	5 trillion ($\sim5 \times 10^{12}$)
<u>0.5% DNA</u>	<u>~46 molecules (~6 feet per cell in total length)</u>
TOTAL	$\sim$100,000 $\times 10^{9}$ or 1×10^{14} (100 trillion) molecules/cell

III. Chemical Reactions/Typical Cell*

Number of enzymes per cell	1-10 billion ($1-10 \times 10^{9}$) enzyme molecules
Total chemical reactions per cell**	billions per minute
DNA replication rates	up to 1000 nucleotide bases per second per cell

* The 200 different cell types in the human body display a significant difference in size, composition, and enzymatic activity.

** Assuming only 25% of the enzymes are active at some level or another

(Thomas C. Spelsberg, 2012)

(2)   Our Cells are Massive Chemical Factories

Equally impressive is the number of chemical (enzymatic) reactions ongoing every minute in one single cell. Enzymes are proteins that speed up chemical reactions over a million fold. The 10 billion or so enzyme molecules per cell catalyze enormous numbers of chemical reactions every minute. Even though the majority of enzyme molecules are not catalyzing at full capacity, and some not active, it has been estimated that in any given minute in one human cell, there can be millions to billions to trillions of ongoing enzymatic reactions! The exact number is unknown, but it must be enormous. The DNA replication enzymes (DNA polymerases) alone can place thousands of single molecules (nucleotides) in a DNA chain every second. If this polymerase enzyme was enlarged to the size of a 6 foot tall person, this would be equivalent to a person travelling down the highway at 600 mph, laying down 4 foot blocks. A typical cell will synthesize 13 million proteins per minute, each with their linear array of amino acids. If one multiplies the 10 billion enzymes per cell by the hundreds of enzyme reactions per minute, and that value by the 10 trillion cells/human body, one obtains a rough estimate of approximately 10^{22} to 10^{28} chemical reactions per minute in each human. These values certainly give one a better appreciation of the complexity and vast numbers of chemical reactions ongoing in each human body.

These numbers above are truly astronomical and give an appreciation as to the complexity (micro-universe) of our individual cells and our bodies, both in terms of its components, and its chemical reactions. As discussed later in Chapter 7, the 20,000 or so protein coding genes in our genome (DNA) code for approximately 100,000 different proteins, each of which interact with each other to create millions of possible combinations/functions. Now we know that a much larger portion of our genome is active, functionally producing RNA molecules, which are involved in regulating when and how much of each of the protein coding genes are expressed (discussed in more detail in Chapter 6). This process gives enormous possible variations. Is it any wonder that scientists have a difficult task and encounter slow progress sifting through this enormous complexity to discover how we get sick, and how to regulate the system to heal our bodies?

D.   The Ultrastructure of Human Cells

How all these molecules are organized and function together inside the human cell are well described in many biology books, but are worth briefly describing here. As figure 4.2 illustrates, the multitude of molecules in a cell are organized into specific subcellular structures, each with specific functions, including membranes, organelles (vesicles surrounded by membranes), cytoskeleton, and more. These structures are the same in cells of all living organisms, including algae, yeast, insect, mammal, plant, and birds (with the exception of bacteria).

Starting from outside the cell and traveling into the cell, we first encounter the dual layer "plasma membrane," which surrounds the entire cell itself, and contains many billions of lipids, proteins, and glycoproteins. There are thousands of different proteins expressed in any given cell membrane. Some of these serve as receptors that bind external signaling molecules such as hormones and growth factors. These communicate the appropriate signals (i.e., messages) within cells and between cells. The cell membrane proteins also serve as cell to cell recognition (coupling) sites, as well as transporters of large molecules through the membrane. The plasma membrane is more fluid than solid with molecular components migrating around it. For example, the lipid molecules can move swiftly around the outer membranes of cells. This migration from one side of a cell to the opposite side has been measured as fast as 15 minutes. If all sizes and distances were made relevant to a lipid molecule which is the height of a six foot tall person, this rapid movement would be equivalent to the person (lipid molecule) traveling at several hundred miles an hour. It is also astonishing that the lipid and protein molecules in the plasma membrane of many of our cells are completely recycled (replaced with new molecules) every four to six hours.

The major internal structures of cells are also shown in figure 4.2. In the cytoplasm, there are other membrane surrounding structures similar to the whole cell membrane. There is the smooth endoplasmic reticulum. The latter is involved in drug and sugar metabolism, the folding and maturation of proteins, including the binding of sugars and lipids to proteins, and the transport of these proteins to various places within the cell, including exportation out of the cell. Another structure is the rough endoplasmic reticulum which contains membrane bound ribosomes and is involved in protein synthesis, processing and protein exportation. It is also involved in cellular transport of proteins, lipids, and sugars. Another structure is the "Golgi apparatus" which is involved in membrane synthesis as well as further processing, packaging, and storage of proteins and lipid products for export out of the cell. In total, the intracellular membranes of a cell are so compact that those in one human liver alone, if spread out as a single bilayer membrane, are estimated to cover six football fields (or 10,000 meters^2). Also found in the cytoplasm are small round packages of protein and RNA called ribosomes. There can be approximately 200,000 of these per cell. These structures synthesize proteins to be utilized inside the cells using the information coded in the

Figure 4.2

Function and Structural Complexity of the Cell

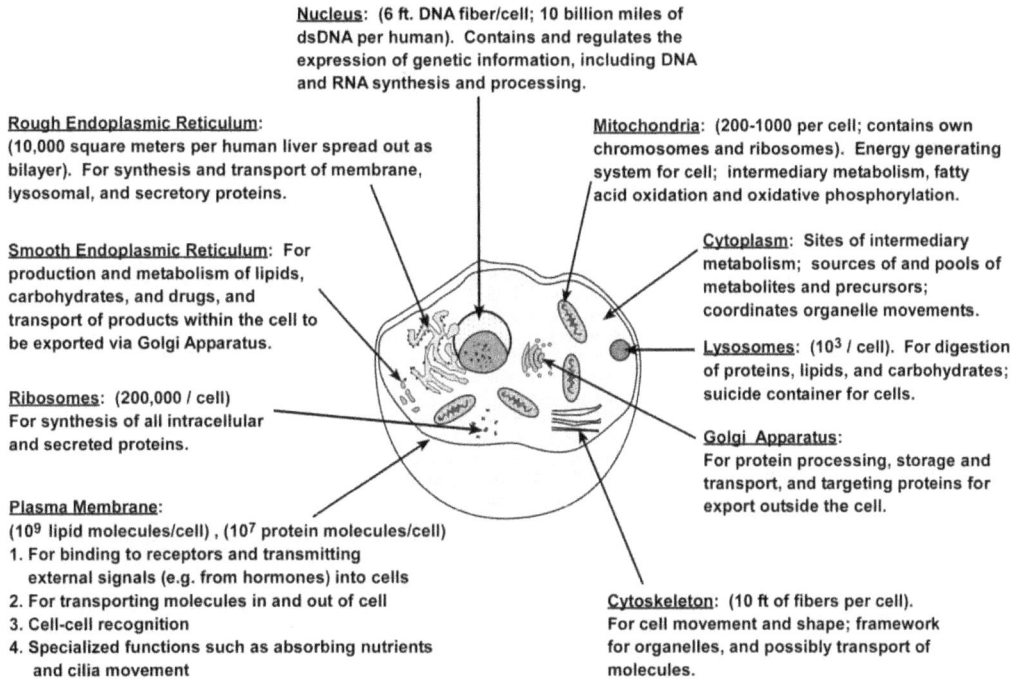

Nucleus: (6 ft. DNA fiber/cell; 10 billion miles of dsDNA per human). Contains and regulates the expression of genetic information, including DNA and RNA synthesis and processing.

Rough Endoplasmic Reticulum:
(10,000 square meters per human liver spread out as bilayer). For synthesis and transport of membrane, lysosomal, and secretory proteins.

Mitochondria: (200-1000 per cell; contains own chromosomes and ribosomes). Energy generating system for cell; intermediary metabolism, fatty acid oxidation and oxidative phosphorylation.

Smooth Endoplasmic Reticulum: For production and metabolism of lipids, carbohydrates, and drugs, and transport of products within the cell to be exported via Golgi Apparatus.

Cytoplasm: Sites of intermediary metabolism; sources of and pools of metabolites and precursors; coordinates organelle movements.

Ribosomes: (200,000 / cell) For synthesis of all intracellular and secreted proteins.

Lysosomes: (10^3 / cell). For digestion of proteins, lipids, and carbohydrates; suicide container for cells.

Golgi Apparatus:
For protein processing, storage and transport, and targeting proteins for export outside the cell.

Plasma Membrane:
(10^9 lipid molecules/cell) , (10^7 protein molecules/cell)
1. For binding to receptors and transmitting external signals (e.g. from hormones) into cells
2. For transporting molecules in and out of cell
3. Cell-cell recognition
4. Specialized functions such as absorbing nutrients and cilia movement

Cytoskeleton: (10 ft of fibers per cell). For cell movement and shape; framework for organelles, and possibly transport of molecules.

(T.C. Spelsberg and K.D. Peters 2011)

messenger RNAs which, in turn, receive their code from the nuclear DNA (genes).

Also shown in figure 4.2, inside each cell one also encounters 50 to 100s of large organelles (the number depends on the cell type and energy demands), termed mitochondria. Mitochondria are surrounded by bilayer lipid membranes and contain their own circular DNA chromosome. Mitochondria multiply and maintain their own population in our cells by undergoing their own divisions, depending on the demand. Each mitochondrion contains 100,000 bundles of enzymes which generate most of the energy for the cell. This energy is in the form of chemical bonds in molecules such as the molecule called "ATP." Each mitochondria has one circular chromosome which replicates and expresses its genes in a process closely resembling that of bacteria (i.e., prokaryote cells). As discussed in Chapter 3, scientists believe that mitochondria were originally bacteria, which at approximately 1.8–2.6 billion years ago, established a symbiotic relationship with other bacteria to create the early eukaryote cells. High doses of antibiotics, which are structured to "poison" only bacteria, often make humans sick, not only by disturbing our microbiome living within us (see Chapter 5), but because they poison the bacterial-like mitochondria inside each of our cells.

Mitochondrial DNA have rapid rates of genetic changes (mutations) that are used by geneticists and anthropologists to study human diseases and trace ancestry. Some mutations on this DNA are known to create inherited (genetic) diseases in humans, including the premature death of infants. Since mitochondria are only transmitted by females via eggs (sperm mitochondria do not enter eggs during fertilization), the female ancestry and female (maternal) related genetic diseases are uniquely traceable to this mitochondrial DNA. It is the Y chromosome in males passed only from father to son, which allows geneticists and anthropologists to track male lineages (i.e., ancestry). These aspects are discussed later in Chapter 7.

Finally, pervading throughout the cell are structures resembling the steel girders of a building (see figure 4.2). These are microfilaments and microtubules forming the cytoskeleton of the cell. This structure is responsible for maintaining cell shape, cell movement, or shape changes, and subcellular structural integrity. This structure is also involved in transporting molecules around the cell. If they are laid end to end, there is an estimated approximately 10 feet of cytoskeletal fibers per cell. Multiplying this value by 10 trillion cells in the human body reveals approximately 20 billion miles of cytoskeleton threads within the human body. These fantastic lengths in a cell are only possible because of the extremely small width of these fibers.

Finally, there is the largest and most visible membrane bound organelle in cells, the nucleus. It contains the chromosomes which contain the genetic information stored in the DNA which code for proteins and RNA to carry out cellular functions. The total chromosomes in each cell contain the genetic information to create a whole human. These structures, and their genetic information together, are called the genome, which is discussed in more detail in Chapter 7.

E.   Cells in Action: Smelling, Walking, and Communicating with Each Other

It is interesting to ponder that certain eukaryote cells in our bodies, and most unicellular organisms, can display physical activities found in multicellular organisms. Believe it or not, some of our cells can walk (i.e., are mobile). They can also smell, eat, and, you might say, defecate (i.e., go to the bathroom). The macrophage and white blood cells are good examples. Macrophages and white blood cells can walk/crawl via "feet" called pseudopodia and even eat by processes known as endocytosis and absorption. This action utilizes structures inside cells, called microfilaments, with mechanical actions resembling our muscle-skeletal system.

More amazing is the fact that the trillions of cells in our bodies work together to coordinate our body functions and activities. This is achieved by a series of communication signals and feedback mechanisms which keep each cell's, and whole body's, processes in balance. Our nervous system and endocrine system (hormones) are part of this whole body communication network to maintain this even balance. In addition, most of our cells secrete and respond to multiple different types of protein chemical messengers, called growth factors or cytokines, which act locally on neighboring cells, and long distances on organs. Other cells secrete endocrine/neurologic hormones which act both locally and distantly on organs and cells. In addition, some of our cells can smell using chemical messages, and their membrane receptors, as do bacteria, and migrate towards or away from the chemical. Macrophages use these agents and their plasma membrane associated specific receptors to detect (sense) the concentrations of these signals in the media around them. The cells then respond by migrating towards the source of these signals, such as bacterial infections and inflammation, to repair these sites. These attractive regulatory agents are classified as cytokines, hormones, or growth factors.

F.   The Coordinated Enormity of it All

In conclusion, we now know that our bodies are an extremely well organized, coordinated mega-community of trillions of small cell micro-universes. How it all works is simply amazing. The regulation of the biochemical pathways coordinates each cell's internal functions. Combining this with the interactive/modulating signals from cell to cell and the communications between the trillions of cells in the tissues of the whole human body, yields enormous complexity. Our bodies coordinate the trillions of cells and tissues via our neurological and endocrine networks. More locally, our cells communicate with each other by growth factors and cytokines and the recently elucidated extracellular "exosomes". The latter are small membrane vesicles containing biologically active DNA, proteins, and RNAs which are secreted by donor cells and enter neighboring cells to alter their activities. Cells also use membrane extensions called "cytonemes," which attach to other cells and exchange signals and possibly chemical substances. It should be mentioned that varying patterns of proteins, lipids, and sugars on our cell membranes are cell type, animal, and human individually specific. This explains immune incompatibility with tissue transplantation. It is no wonder that progress in medical science seems "slow," and so difficult. With the above in mind, the medical/biological achievements have been amazingly rapid, even though the human cells and body are as complex as the cosmos. When we add the massive load of bacteria in our bodies (the human microbiome) (discussed in the following two chapters) with approximately 10 living bacteria cells for every one of our cells, this complexity increases still further.

Section II

The Human Microbiome and our Health

(The Bacteria within Us)

Chapter 5

The Microbial World: Vast Numbers and a Symbiotic Social Life with Higher Life Forms

Definitions

bacterial (bio-) films: a community of microbes of different species attached to a surface and functioning in a symbiotic relationship; slimy appearance (e.g., dental plaque).

extremophiles: any microbe (bacteria, fungi, protists) that inhabits extreme environments (e.g., heat, salt, acidity, pressure); they usually use chemical elements for energy and breathing.

microbes: microscopic organisms consisting of bacteria, viruses, or protists (e.g., prokaryote and eukaryote); many are pathogenic.

microbiome: population of microbes (viruses, bacteria, protists, spirochetes, and fungi) inhabiting in and on the human body.

quorum sensing: phenomenon in which a population of bacteria produces and responds to intercellular chemical signals whose concentration indicates the density and the species of the cellular population nearby; their genes often respond to these signals in order to relate symbiotically and coordinate their actions for mutual benefit of the community.

symbiosis: kingdoms, phyla, and species living together in permanent or prolonged close association with mutual benefits for both species (e.g., bacterial plaques and biofilms).

A.   The Massive Population and Complexity of the Bacteria World

   (1)   Introduction and Whole Earth Populations

We have all heard about microbes: We have especially heard about the pathological microbes that make us sick. This chapter discusses the world of these micro-organisms: their resilience, amazing diversity, and astounding numbers. The term "microbes" represents several kingdoms: Bacteria (prokaryotes), Fungi (eukaryotes), and protista (single celled) organisms with nuclei (which are also eukaryotes). Chapters 5 and 6 focus on bacteria, since they predominate the microbes in and on humans. Bacteria live everywhere on the surface of the earth, including in a symbiotic relationship with almost all multicellular organisms including humans. These bacteria represent the human microbiome: they reside primarily on our skin, in our orifices, and in our intestines.

As discussed in Chapter 3 and summarized in table 5.1, bacteria are the largest class of biomass on Earth, and represent the first living organisms on Earth. They represent over half of all the Earth's biomass. Bacteria live to eat and divide (reproduce). What many people do not know is that humans, like all other multicellular animals (e.g., mammals, fish, and insects), as well as fungi and plants, harbor large numbers of bacteria that live in a symbiotic relationship with their bodies. As discussed earlier, bacteria appeared on Earth 3.8–4.0 billion years ago, shortly after the earth cooled, hardened, and was almost completely covered by oceans. They represent the oldest life on Earth. They even appeared to survive the massive asteroid and comet bombardment that occurred 3.8–4.2 billion years ago, and might even have been brought to Earth by these extraterrestrial bodies. Approximately 2-3 billion years ago, cyanobacteria first used photosynthesis to give Earth its atmospheric oxygen, which is so vital to life today. Eubacteria and

Archaea represent the two domains (subkingdoms) of the bacteria (prokaryote) family surviving today. They outnumber all other life forms on Earth with a population estimated at 5×10^{31} individuals (i.e., 50 x million x trillion x trillion) out of an Earth total of approximately 10^{33} living organisms. Combined, Earth's bacteria weigh approximately 50×10^{15} (i.e., 50 x million x billion or 50 quadrillion) tons representing over half of the planet's biomass. If all the bacteria on Earth are placed end to end, they would stretch approximately 1×10^{23} miles (i.e., 100 x billion x trillion miles), or 80% of the distance from Earth to the edge of the visible universe (table 5.1).

New genomic (RNA) analyses are now being used to identify different bacteria species, which is far superior to the old cell culturing methods, especially since many bacteria cannot be cultured in the laboratory. The term "species," until recently, was a biological classification used to distinguish groups of bacteria that appeared similar to each other in lab culture plates. Today, the species are classified by molecular genetics. This new technique, using metagenomics technology involving the sequencing of ribosomal RNA, is termed "molecular phylogenomics." It is now estimated that 30–150 million (30–150 x 10^6) species of bacteria are living on Earth. Some scientists even estimate that there are as many as ten billion (10^{10}) species living on the earth. It should be mentioned that even more novel sequencing technologies have evolved to more accurately distinguish distinct species of bacteria, and identifying their biological functions: e.g., "metagenomics," "single amplified genomes (SAGs)," "multiple displacement amplification (MDA)," "linear thermal cycling amplification," and "Malbac". Using

Table 5.1

General Facts about Bacteria
(prokaryotes/archea)

1. Bacteria, e.g. archea at 0.3-10 microns long and nanobacteria at .050-0.20 microns long, vastly outnumber all other life forms on earth at 5 x10^{31} (50 million x trillion x trillion) strong. Most are yet unidentified. There are an estimated 5 x 10^7 species.

2. They have been around for 3.8-4.0 billion years, and are believed to be the oldest life form.

3. Some can reproduce in 10 minutes, thus going from 1 cell to a billion in 5 hours. They live to reproduce and eat.

4. Bacteria represent half of the planets biomass.

5. Lined up end to end, earth's bacteria would stretch 10 billion light years (~ 10^{23} miles), i.e., 80% of the distance to the edge of the visible universe.

(Thomas C. Spelsberg, 2012)

these techniques, it has been found that most species of bacteria (approximately 99.999%) have never been identified or classified.

(2)   The Oceans

It has been estimated that 9 out of 10 living species on Earth, including bacteria, live in the ocean waters and ocean floor. The ocean waters alone harbor hundreds of millions of species of microbes, but currently only 230,000 have names and 95% are unknown. Based on direct samplings of the ocean waters, scientists estimate that about 1 billion bacteria are present in each drop of ocean water. About 10^{30} new bacteria cells are produced (replenished by bacterial cell divisions) each year just on the ocean surface waters. That number is estimated to exceed the number of individual grains of sand on the entire earth by a factor of 10 billion fold. One estimate calculates that there is at least 145 billion tons of bacteria in the 320 million cubic miles of water covering Earth's 140 million square miles of ocean. An even greater number live on and below the ocean floor. Some microbiologists estimate that 40% of the earth's bacteria reside in the ocean floor alone.

(3)   The Atmosphere

Live bacteria have even been found floating in our atmosphere as high as 60,000–80,000 feet at temperatures of -50°F. Up to 2 million tons (4 billion pounds) of bacteria along with approximately 100 billion tons of fungal spores are estimated to be blown into the earth's atmosphere each year. Recent studies have found large numbers of bacteria in the jet stream, wherein an estimated 5100 bacteria per cubic meter of air are found at 10 kilometers elevation. These are living and reproducing bacteria that feed on organic chemicals in the air. It is hypothesized that airborne bacteria trigger most of the rain drops in storms. One wonders if these airborne bacteria are blown into outer space by solar wind, possibly spreading life to other worlds. Bacteria have been found on rocket ships, satellites, and planetary probes, and survived on these objects for years in the vacuum and extreme temperatures of space.

B.   The Size of Bacteria

Also listed in table 5.1 and depicted in figure 3.2, a typical human eukaryotic cell measures 10–50 microns in diameter, while most bacteria measure 10–50 times smaller (0.2–2.0) microns in diameter, which is approximately 5×10^{-5} of an inch or 5 one hundred thousandths of an inch. Overall, bacteria sizes vary over 5000 fold. The smallest bacteria, called nano-bacteria, have a diameter approximately 10 times smaller than most bacteria (less than 0.1 micron), while a few larger species of bacteria can reach the eukaryotic cell size (approximately 20 microns diameter). The average bacteria are extremely small, about 1/10–1/50 the size of our own cells. A colony of average sized bacteria (3 inch diameter), residing on a flat surface, contains 600 billion bacteria, 100 times more than there are humans (6 billion) on Earth. There are more than one billion bacteria in a teaspoon of yogurt and an estimated trillion (10^{12}) bacteria in a teaspoon of garden soil, representing about 10,000 species.

Figure 5.1 shows a picture of a probiotic pill, used to calm our intestines, which is smaller than a dime and sold over the counter. Each small pill contains 500 million (half a billion, i.e., 500,000,000 or 5×10^{8}) bacteria. This gives a good perspective that bacteria are really small. Bacteria are survivors, surviving extremes of environment and rapidly reproducing. Some bacteria can divide every 10 minutes, going from one cell to a billion cells in 5 hours. To give you a real picture of what some different species of bacteria look like, figure 5.2 shows an electron microscopic photo of human gut bacteria at 10,000 x magnification containing a few different species of the 1000 or so total different species found in our intestines.

C.   Bacteria Live Everywhere: Many are Extremophiles

As outlined in table 5.2, bacteria, called extremophiles, can exist miles below the earth's crust, deep in the ocean, below the ocean floor, around ocean vents, in and on rocks at Earth's poles, inside glaciers, and in our intestines. Some bacteria "eat" and survive on minerals and water. Others even eat poisons (e.g., arsenic), as well as oil and other organic solvents. Bacteria have no specific life span, and in short, are immortal. Their sole purpose is to survive and reproduce. Some bacteria, lying in hibernation over 2–3 miles deep in the earth, have survived millions of years and shown to be alive as they can be cultured and grown in the laboratory. The oldest recorded living oxygen breathing bacteria have been estimated to be 86 million years old, exhibiting very low metabolism, and living in clay one-half mile deep below the ocean floor. Hibernating live bacteria have even been found inside rocks that are 4 billion years old. Their age was not estimated. Hibernating bacteria, originating on NASA engineers and our astronauts of Apollo 12, have even survived on the moon for over 3 years, exposed to temperature extremes of -250°F to +250°F with solar radiation and no atmosphere.

Some extremophiles are found in the rocks and permafrost of Arctic and dry Antarctic valleys at -15°C (similar to the planet Mars) and deep in the earth at pressures of up to 5000 atmospheres (75,000 pounds per square inch). A tablespoon of mud from 11,000 meters deep in the ocean floor was found to contain 10 million bacteria. Extremophiles are also found near hydrothermal vents

Figure 5.1

The Size of Bacteria

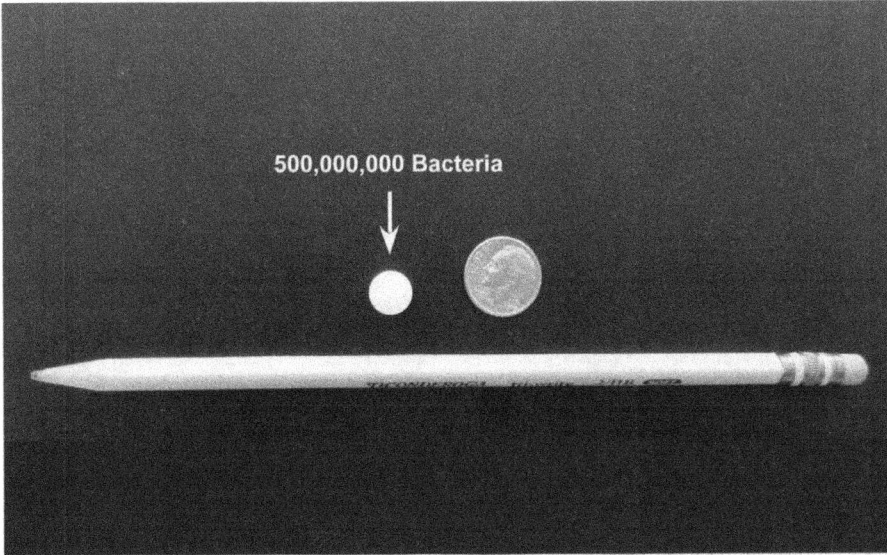

(T. Spelsberg & K. Peters, 2012)

Figure 5.2

Representative Human Intestinal Flora of the 1000+ Species of Bacteria

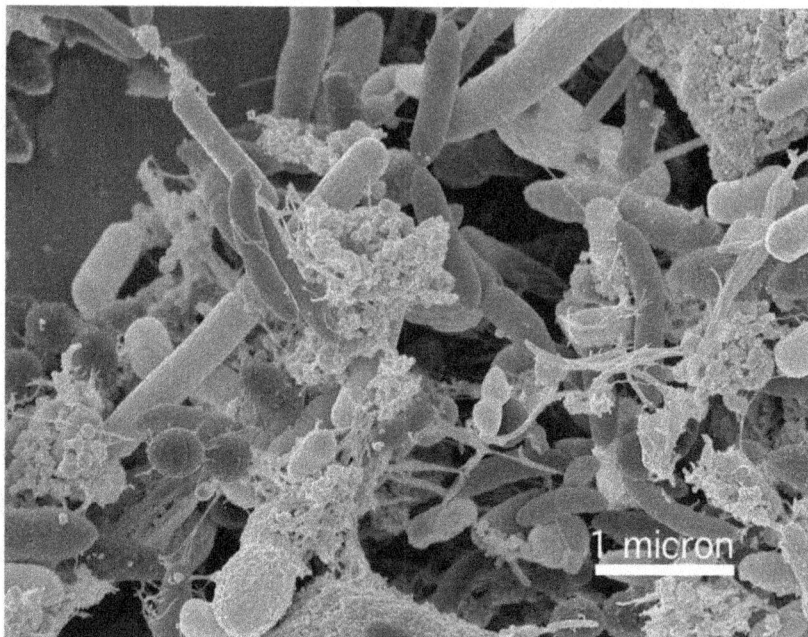

Courtesy of Christina Schwach, Talmud Torah High School, St Paul, MN and Dr. Jeffrey L. Salisbury, Mayo Clinic, Rochester, MN. (10,000 X magnification)

Figure 5.2. Representative human 10,000 x (power) intestinal flora of the 1000+ species of bacteria.
Courtesy of Dr. Tina Schwach (Talmud Torah High School) and Dr. Jeff Salisbury (Mayo Clinic).

Table 5.2

Extremophiles Bacteria at the Extremes (archea)

- **Cold (Psychrophiles):** live below freezing temperatures (-15 °C). Ice (including glaciers) in Antarctica has huge numbers of "living" bacteria (trillions, 10^{13}), some 8 million years old, which are still alive (i.e., can be cultured) *(Dark Life, M. Taylor, 1999).*

- **Heat (Thermophiles):** live above boiling temp (212-500 °F).

- **Salt (Halophiles):** live in water 100 x saltier than the ocean.

- **Acid (Acidophiles):** live at pH below 1.0.

- **Alkali (Alkaliphiles):** live at pH >9.0.

- **Pressure (Barophiles):** live 2 miles below the Earth, 7 miles deep in the ocean, and 0.5 miles below the sea floor. Some are estimated to be 86 million years old.

- **Dry (Xerophiles):** live without water.

- **No Oxygen (Anaerobes):** live without air/oxygen.

(Thomas C. Spelsberg, 2012)

on the deep ocean floor, where the temperature (>130°F) and pressure (>1,000 atmospheres or approximately 15,000 pounds per square inch) resemble that of the planet Venus.

Other extremophiles live away from vents at below freezing temperatures and at huge pressures, while some live in oxygen-free conditions (e.g., deep in the earth or in our intestines). Recent studies in Antarctica identified living bacteria (approximately 10,000 per tablespoon) in Lake Whillans and Lake Vostok, 800 meters and 4000 meters, respectively, below the ice sheet. These bacteria have been isolated for millions of years from the rest of our world. Interestingly, evidence of multicellular eukaryote aquatic organisms (e.g., insects and zooplankton) have also been identified in these lake waters.

Extremophiles can live in solutions 100 times saltier than the ocean, in very acidic conditions (pH below 1.0), or in very alkaline conditions (above 9.0 pH). Thus, microbes (bacteria and archaea) are survivors, surviving at much broader salt, acid, and alkali environments, and at temperatures and pressures which are too extreme for other life forms. For the chemist in all of us, scientists have now learned that extremophiles survived by having mutations in many of their proteins, that allowed them to operate normally under extreme conditions. For example, those who thrive in strong acids or alkali have stabilized (cross-linked) protein chains. Those who thrive in cold conditions have less charge on their protein surfaces and more chain flexibility, reducing their interactions with water. This permits normal functioning in the cold. Those in high salt and hot conditions have many negative groups on their protein surfaces to keep a shell of pure water around them.

In addition to the photosynthesis and oxygen based respiration system, some extremophiles, called anaerobes, use oxidized inorganic molecules/ elements, which are useless to other living organisms, for respiration and energy. Examples of these are nitrates, hydrogen sulfide, methane, ammonia, iron, etc., (see table 5.3). Overall, 90% of life in the high salt waters are microbes (halophiles), representing both single eukaryote cell plants (phytoplankton) and extremophile bacteria. Extremophile microbes (mainly bacteria) are the master recyclers on the earth. They feed on the dead plankton, fish, excrement, and whatever falls to the depths of the ocean floor, as well as whatever plants, animals, or insects that die on land. They decompose this organic material and secrete the generated organic molecules (usually with bad odors) for other life forms to use.

D.   Bacteria Living with Other Living Organisms (Symbiosis)

Not all bacteria are "bad" for human health. In fact, many live in harmony with us (our human microbiome) and give us good health and protect us. Bacteria often work symbiotically with each other and with their much larger hosts, including animals, plants, insects, and humans (discussed in detail in the next chapter). Symbiosis is when two different species work together to better survive. In this role, each species serves important physiological or protective functions for the other. Symbiosis occurs all over the earth among all species. Symbiosis occurs between bacteria and most other multicellular organisms (animals, plants, insects, and fungi) on Earth, including termites and tubeworms at the bottom of the ocean, all mammals, insects, many plants, and humans (see next chapter). Keep in mind that not all organisms live together symbiotically. Some combinations are parasitic

Table 5.3

Extremophile Respiration

- The extremophiles utilize various forms of respiration from photosynthesis and aerobic respiration to anaerobic respiration. As the depths in the earth and ocean increase, the anaerobic extremophiles utilize - in order: NO_3 Mn, Fe, SO_4 and even H_2 .
  (DeLong - Science, 301, Dec. 2004)

- Some extremophiles produce methane, concentrate gold from water, and even digest oil and other organic molecules / solvents.
  (See book lists for: D. Wharton, 2002, Life at the Limits; M. Taylor, 1999, Dark Life; M. Gross, 1996, Life on the Edge; T. Gold, 1999, The Deep Hot Biosphere; C. Needham et al, 2000, "Intimate Strangers: Unseen Life on Earth"

(Thomas C. Spelsberg, 2012)

whereby only one of the pair benefits, the other organism is usually hurt by the dweller.

All mammals live in a symbiotic relationship with bacteria. The most well known are cows, horses, rhinos, and other ruminants, discussed below. Life is smart – doing whatever it takes to survive. Combinations of many different species of bacteria usually live symbiotically within host organisms: communicating via chemical messages with each other and with the cells of the host. In large bacterial films (e.g., dental plaques), each species (of the many) contributes and receives nutrients and protection from the group as a whole: a true socialistic society. Using chemical signals, many of which bind to receptors on their membranes, they can determine the presence of their own species as well as other species in their neighborhood, including which species is friend or which is foe. In this process, known as "Quorum Sensing," bacteria use these cell surface "identifier"/receptors and chemical "factors" secreted by each member to communicate with others in the colony as a whole about who is around (i.e., neighbors). These chemical messengers are further described in the next section.

Plants sequester carbon dioxide from the air to synthesize organic compounds using photosynthesis; however, they cannot sequester nitrogen from the earth, which is also needed by the plants for survival. Their required nitrogen is obtained by symbiotic bacteria (rhizobium) or the fungi (mycorrhizae); both sequester nitrogen at the plant roots, and share the nitrogen with the plants in exchange for carbon-based nutrients such as sugars and amino acids. As a reminder, fungi are single or multicellular organisms comprised of eukaryote cells, i.e., the type of cells with nuclei and mitochondria or chloroplasts that make up "higher" organisms such as animals and plants, respectively. Fungi and bacteria also help plants extract minerals and water from the soil. They also protect plants from pathogens and toxic wastes.

The gut bacteria in insects provide essential amino acids to aphids and supply B vitamins to the tsetse fly. They also help digest wood in the termite. In the animal world, the large vegetarians, such as goats, cows, camels, giraffes, rhinos, elephants, etc., called ruminants, have four separate compartments in their stomachs. Two of the compartments contain biofilms comprised of hundreds of trillions of bacteria of many species, mostly extremophiles of the phylum, archaea, and eukaryote organisms such as protozoa and fungi. These symbiotic gut organisms have enzymes that digest plant cellulose into energy, sugars, and other nutrients. Something similar to this occurs in humans, although to a lesser extent, and is discussed in the next chapter. It is interesting that recent genomic analyses have demonstrated support for "horizontal gene transfer" between different symbiotic organisms, such as bacteria, fungi, algae, and their hosts, which allows them to share their genes and thus their various metabolic attributes.

E.   More about the Chemical Communications, Competition, and Locomotion among Bacteria

Communities of mixed bacteria types (different species) are always in communication with each other via "quorum sensing" and allow the whole bacterial community to know who is around, friend or foe. In this manner, they work as a "society" in our intestines to help keep us healthy. This communication is achieved via secreted factors that bind to the cell membranes of neighboring bacteria or via cell to cell contact with nearby bacteria. Examples of known bacterial paracrine communicators (See Chapter 11) are peptides/proteins, surfactins, peptoglycans, protein cytokines, growth factors, and metabolites, e.g., benzoate and sugars. The bacteria paracrine communicators are either "attractants," "repellants," or communicators as to who is around. Receptors on the surface of bacteria bind these signals either to elicit aggregation/attraction or to connect (anchor) the two cells together. Interesting examples of these signaling communicators are the proteins that can signal bacteria to aggregate for protection purposes or to increase certain aspects of their metabolism. Some factors are "alert" messages: signaling the presence of enemy bacteria. Once signaled, many will combat these enemy cells with toxins and some will even commit suicide to protect the community as a whole. Other communicators serve as signals for regulating the production of needed nutrients among the population. As mentioned above, the concentrations of some of these factors are now known to serve as sensors of the population size, as well as identifying which species of bacteria are living in the population. In short, this communication helps the whole community work more efficiently as one – once a signal is received, bacteria are known to respond within milliseconds (thousandths of a second) and some bacteria are able to travel 10–20 bacteria cell lengths per second towards or away from these chemical signals. This is really fast. As a means of moving around, bacteria use appendages like cilia, wiggling, flapping of the membrane, and chemical-receptor interactions on their surfaces.

F.   Devious Actions of Pathogenic Bacteria

Pathogenic organisms which make us (and other living organisms) sick, however, have learned devious plans to take advantage of the communications among the good (symbiotic) bacteria community. These "bad"/pathogenic bacteria "eavesdrop" on these chemical messages and have learned to block and even mimic these signals so they can "take personal advantage of" or eliminate the competing population of good bacteria. Some pathogenic bacteria enter the cells of our bodies (and those of other animals, and insects) and proliferate. Some will produce toxins which make the host sick, further assisting the survival of the bad bacteria. Some pathogenic bacteria have developed tactics to invade other bacterial cells. Using this defense, they multiply to re-infect additional bacterial cells, to ultimately taking over the good, symbiotic bacteria. An example is *Salmanella typhi* which causes typhoid fever. This bacterium multiplies and invades neighboring bacterial cells, further enhancing the illness in the human host. Others, such as *Helicobacter pylori* and *Clostridium difficile*, create intestinal disorders by producing toxins to kill and then devour the good symbiotic bacteria, as well as irritating and killing our own human (eukaryotic) cells. As will be discussed in the following chapter, our bodies constantly exchange chemical messages with our symbiotes of the microbial world (bad and good) which reside in our bodies (our microbiome) to identify "friend or foe," a phenomenon sometimes called "interkingdom signaling."

Chapter 6

The Human Microbiome and Our Health: The Massive Bacterial World within Us

Definitions

dysbiosis: imbalances in the microbiome associated with human diseases and ailments.

horizontal gene transfer: transfer of genetic information from one species to another, as they live side by side.

inflammatory cytokines: paracrine or hormonal proteins secreted mainly by macrophages involved in encouraging inflammation to combat diseases, pathogens, or abnormal tissues (cancer calcified tissues, such as heart valves); examples are interleukin 1, tumor necrosis factor, leukotrienes, fatty acids, and lipopolysaccharides; some of these are secreted by damaged tissues.

International Human Microbiome Consortium: a multinational organizational/ institutional consortium, collaborating to determine all the species of bacteria living in and on humans at various body locations.

pathogenic bacteria: also called "bad" bacteria or disease-causing bacteria.

pathogens: any disease causing parasite – bacterial, viral, fungal, or protozoa.

probiotics: substances (foods/yogurt or pills) containing bacterial populations beneficial for the digestive system that help maintain a healthy digestive system by combating pathogenic bacteria.

A.   Introduction and Overview

This chapter discusses the myriad of bacteria that reside on and inside humans. Humans depend on bacteria for survival and our health. For further reading on the human microbiome, see the "References for Further Reading" section for this chapter, especially the new book by Arrange, et al, 2013. Our human microbiome can be viewed as an independent organ. Initially acquired at birth (via the birth canal), they help steer our development, immune system, and metabolic pathways for energy storage and consumption. C-section babies, unfortunately, fail to get much of this benefit. As discussed in the previous chapter, humans, like all animals, insects, and plants, have evolved an essential symbiotic relationship with microbes. This symbiosis probably began 2 to 3 billion years ago among different bacterial species and continued 500 million to one billion years ago among early multicellular animals, including mammals (60 million years ago).

As outlined in table 6.1, the human body harbors a huge multitude of colonies of bacteria, both inside and outside the body, adding up to about 10 bacteria for every 1 of our human cells. This value represents a total of approximately 100 trillion (10^{14}) bacteria in and on each human. These bacteria are currently being identified by molecular analyses, "molecular phylogenomics," described in Chapter 5, as most cannot be grown in the lab. These bacteria that reside in humans represent the "human microbiome." The combination of all the genes of the total human microbiome contains over 1000 times the genetic information (approximately 300 million different genes) than our own genome. Each human appears to have approximately 8 million bacterial genes compared to our human 22,000 genes. We now know they help us digest our foods, regulate our weight and immune system, affect our moods including our sense of well-being, keep pathogens (bad bacteria) at bay, and prepare us for the world when we are first born.

The International Human Microbiome Consortium (IHMC) which was launched in 2007 has been organized to examine the human microbiome of 250 humans at a cost of $170 million. It has the following two goals: 1) to identify as many species of bacteria in and on the human body of a multitude of people, and 2) to understand their role in human health and disease. Over $160 million has been spent as of 2012 on this project, focusing on approximately 4800 samples from 5 areas of the human body: nasopharyngeal, gastrointestinal, oral cavity, skin, and female urogenital tracts, as well as stool samples. This accurate, large scale identification of different bacterial species in our intestines and skin is being achieved using "metagenomics" technology in the Human Microbiome Project.

It involves the metagenomic approach using the comparative analyses of ribosomal RNA (rRNA) sequences of each species. This technology is far superior than using the old method of culturing bacteria in the laboratory. To date, the International Human Microbiome Project (IHMP) has identified and analyzed 70 million bacterial rRNA sequences, and 60 million bacterial genes in thousands of healthy human adults. One major discovery has evolved from these studies: a high biodiversity of microbes in our body correlates with good health, and a low diversity correlates with poor health. It appears that a more diverse population of bacteria keeps all species in check, and us healthy. The manipulation of the gut microbiota has helped humans with bowel/intestinal diseases, obesity, mental disposition, and our metabolic syndrome.

As outlined in table 6.1, it is hard to imagine that the human body harbors

Table 6.1

Our Microbiome: The Estimated Total Population of Bacteria in and on the Human Body

Location and Organisms	Estimated Quantity
A. Bacteria cells/human cells in human body	~10 fold (10^{14} or 100 trillion)
B. Percent of human body weight as bacteria	Up to 20%
C. Number of species of bacteria in or on humans	112,000 species
1. Skin (different areas - different species)	Several trillions of bacteria as ~120 different species. Mostly aerobic eubacteria. Women have many more skin bacteria than men.
2. Mouth/teeth	Hundreds of billions of bacteria in dental plaques with a total of ~1000 species found in humans. Individuals have ~160 different species.
3. Hands	Many millions of bacteria with 150 species per individual human and 83% unique to the left or right hands (A sample of 100 people contained a total of 5000 species with 5% common to all hands)
4. Intestine	100 trillion bacteria with the colon containing the most, followed by the intestine and stomach. There are as 35,000 different species, but ~1,000 are predominate, with a combination of eubacteria and ancient anaerobic bacteria (archaea)
D. Biological classifications and distributions of all bacteria found in 10 individuals	19 phyla, 205 genera, 112,000 species
E. Pathogenic (bad) bacteria on humans	~100 species (types)
F. Prominent pathogenic bacteria found in humans	Percent of humans colonized by these pathogenic bacteria.
Mycobacterium causing Tuberculosis/leprosy	35%
Heliobacteria pylori causing stomach ulcers/cancers	50%
Staphylococcus aureus infections of respiratory system and skin wounds	50%
G. Viruses	There are ~10×10^{15} (10 quadrillion) viruses in each human. 100 viruses per bacteria, 1000 viruses per human cell in our bodies. Most invade and live in bacteria, but some live in (infect) our human cells. Many do no harm (that we know of).

(Thomas C. Spelsberg, 2013)

83

an estimated total of 10^{14} (a hundred trillion) bacteria, which means that 9 out of every 10 living cells in our bodies are bacteria, or only one cell out of 10 represents our own cells. There are about a thousand times more bacteria just in your gut alone than the 110 billion humans that ever lived. The total mass of bacteria in and on a human body represents up to 20% of our whole body weight. In essence, we humans are complex biologic "supra-organisms."

Bacteria reside not only on our skin, but also under fingernails and in our mouths, ears, nose, and intestines (see table 6.1). The human microbiome plays a role in our health supported by the fact that the presence of good bacteria in our guts has been shown to be a major force in inhibiting the growth of "bad" bacteria which cause diseases and illnesses. It should be noted that the sweat, blood, lymph, urine, and organs of our bodies normally contain no bacteria before exposure to the environment, i.e., these domains are normally sterile. An unexpected discovery revealed that the composition of any individual's intestinal microbiome is not determined so much by the person's genetics, but rather mostly by diet and environment. Thus, people of different geographic areas differ more in their gut bacteria than people of the same area. Identical twins living together, but with different diets, have different gut microbiomes. This difference becomes greater as the different environments become more diverse. The following sections will discuss the bacteria population in the various parts of our bodies as well as their functions as symbiotes. Together, all of these symbiotic bacteria listed below represent "the human microbiome."

B.   Skin: The Transmitting of Microbes to Others

Recently, just from the skin of 10 individual humans, scientists have identified a total human microbiome of 19 different phyla and 205 genera, totaling more than 112,000 species of bacteria (see table 6.1). Believe it or not, there are about 100,000 bacteria per square centimeter (¼ of square inch) of human skin. That calculates to several trillion on the skin of each human body. One bacterial species, *Staphylococcus*, was the dominant species on the skin of all individuals. The balance of bacterial species populations is unique to individuals. Those on the skin produce specific odors unique for each person, one that dogs can detect. Every time we touch someone or something, we exchange many hundreds of thousands of bacteria. Our pets and any animals we touch also exchange their bacteria with us. It seems scary, but this exchange is usually helpful to our health.

Table 6.2 summarizes the bacterial population on human skin and in mouths. In one study, twenty different sites of the skin from 10 different individuals were recently examined. The same areas among the 10 people harbored somewhat similar, but still unique, populations (species) of bacteria. In contrast, different skin areas of each person's body displayed vastly different (unique) populations. Each of our hands harbors millions of bacteria involving about 150 species (table 6.2). The hands from a hundred individuals were found to contain a total of 4,742 species of bacteria, with only 5 species common to all hands. Interestingly, in all instances, approximately 80% of the bacteria species differed between the left and right hands. This makes sense, as we use our two hands for different functions. After washing thoroughly (which reduces, but doesn't eliminate all the bacteria) and returning a day later, each individual regained the same comparable bacterial populations on their hands that they originally had. This is probably due to the repopulation by the residual population and the individual human's contact with their daily items: their friends, family, clothing, computer, and

<u>Table 6.2</u>

Bacteria and Us

---

1. Each of our bodies harbors 100 trillion (10^{14}) bacteria which is 10 x more than our own cells and represents ~20% of our body weight.

2. On human hands of 50 individuals, 4,742 species of bacteria were found; only 5 species were common to all hands.

3. On average, each hand harbors 150 species, with 83% unique between left and right hands.

4. Women's skin harbor more species and greater number of bacteria than men's.

5. Each human mouth contains 160 species and hundreds of billions of bacteria. A total of 1000 species have been identified in the mouths of the human population examined so far.

other utensils containing the original bacterial population.

The bacterial populations on human skin are so unique to each of us that the bacterial species we leave with our fingers and other body areas that come into contact with various items, are as individually unique as are our fingerprints. Our skin bacteria have recently been shown to play a role in repelling insect bites as well as disease-causing bacteria. This is why some people seem to be less bothered by mosquitoes. Since both our skin cells and the bacteria on them give off odors, animals (dogs) can identify each of us not only by the odors of our human cells, but also the odors from the bacteria on our skin. The odor trail that dogs use to track us is from the skin cells and bacteria that we shed. The 35 million (3.5×10^7) bacteria shed per hour from each of us are only a minor fraction (0.001%) of the 3 to 5 trillion (3-5 $\times 10^{12}$) bacteria on our skin. These bacteria constantly divide to repopulate on the skin. This process occurs elsewhere in our bodies.

It is interesting to note that there is also a gender specificity of skin bacteria populations – with women having a greater number of skin bacteria than men. This is speculated to be due to men's more acidic perspiration and women's growth promoting/nutrient skin cream applications. In contrast, women may have more bacteria on them, but the habitats of men (offices and residences) have been shown to have more microbes than those of women - probably reflecting the better cleanliness of women than men. In the office, phones have the most bacteria, followed by chairs and computer keyboards. At home, the TV remotes, computer keyboards, cell phones, door knobs, light switches, and faucets have the most bacteria. Overall, billions to trillions of bacteria consisting of over 500 different genera and thousands of species of bacteria have been found in our offices and residences, reflecting the bacteria from the skin, mouth, nose, and even bacteria from contaminating traces of feces. The bacterial population in an office or home also depends on the people (and pets) who have visited. The longer the visit of people and pets, the greater the bacteria population found in that room resembles those of the visitor. This is obviously due to the continual shedding of our skin bacteria along with our own skin cells. The allergic house dust has been shown to contain huge numbers of bacteria, largely coming from the 35 million bacteria shed per hour from humans and pets along with millions of skin cells.

It should be noted that most, but not all, of our skin bacteria are good bacteria (i.e., those which cause no health issues) and even help fight off "bad" (pathogenic) bacteria. The bad bacteria are those that cause disease and health issues. One example of the bad bacteria residing on our skin is *Staphylococcus*. When an open wound or surgery occurs on the skin or when we touch the more vulnerable mouth, nose, and eye tissues with "dirty" fingers, we can get "infections" because the bad bacteria on our skin then have an opportunity to invade. A recent major discovery has revealed that it is the good bacteria on our skin that retard the bad bacterial populations from expanding: thus, the good bacteria protect us from bacterial infections and related diseases. Recently, scientists at the University of Pennsylvania reported that lab animals (mice) raised with no skin bacteria displays a reduced immunity against wound and internal infections. This immunity was restored when skin bacteria was replenished. Somehow skin bacteria communicate with the immune system to enhance its readiness to fight future bacterial infections. So, in addition to fighting against bad bacteria, the good skin bacteria enhance our immune response. It should be noted that even "good" bacteria can be deleterious to us if they invade our bodies in normally sterile places in sufficient numbers.

C.   Our Mouth and Tooth Decay

Using the new genomic (DNA) technologies to analyze ribosomal RNA species, the mouths of humans are now known to contain a huge number of different species of bacteria which, when combined, number in the billions of individual bacteria (table 6.1). Most of these are of unknown species. Our tongues have been shown to contain approximately 8,000 species of bacteria, while our noses harbor approximately 2,000 species and throats approximately 4,000 species. The mouth/teeth bacterial colonies are true biofilms, i.e., symbiotic communities of different species of bacteria (and sometimes fungi) working together as "teams", an example of which are the "dental plaques." The populations of these communities vary, depending on what we eat. Each of these small plaques on our teeth contain up to 10 billion (10^{10}) bacteria. Individuals share their mouth bacteria by sharing food and drink, and even more so by open mouth kissing. The new revelation is that we share our bacteria along with our love.

The bacteria in the plaques on our teeth cooperate and compete with each other. To our amazement, they can share their genetic material with each other (termed "horizontal gene transfer"). The bacteria on our teeth that cause decay are primarily "*Streptococcus* mutans" (*S. mutans*) which produce lactic acid from dietary sugars which, in turn, dissolves enamel. These bacteria are followed by *Lactobacillus* which further digests and destroys the teeth. Recent analyses of teeth of prehistoric humans have shown that cavities and the populations of *S. mutans* and related species in the teeth became dominant approximately 10,000 years ago (8000 BC), the time when humans began farming and eating sugar enriched cereal grains. Tooth cavities and bacteria further increased in the 1850s during the industrial revolution when refined sugars entered the diets. Mouth washes and tooth brushing greatly decreases the population of bacteria and reduces lactic acid production and tooth decay, at least for several hours, but do not remove all bacteria. So brush well, as you are fighting billions of reproducing bacteria every day to save your teeth.

D.   The Digestive Tract and Intestinal Diseases

(1)   Introduction

The largest population of bacteria in the human body and in other animals (e.g., mammals, insects, amphibians, birds, and fish), resides in the stomach and intestines. They live in a symbiotic relationship with us and with each other. Most of these bacteria are anaerobic extremophiles of the "Archaea" domain (phylum) (see figure 3.1). As summarized in table 6.3, a human GI tract has up to 100 trillion (10^{14}) bacteria, a few reside in the acidic (hydrochloric acid) stomach, more in the small intestine (approximately 10^5 to 10^6 per millimeter of fluid), but most (95%) reside in the large intestine. Most (approximately 60% to 70%) of the suspected 35,000 species of bacteria that exist in the global human intestines are unknown. There is an estimated 1000 species in any individual human gut. Our gut bacteria are attached to the intestinal cells either through a glue they produce or via specific proteins on the outer cell membranes of bacteria that bind to our intestinal cells. It appears that we obtain our first GI microbes from our mothers, during passage through the birth canal and subsequently from breast feeding. Therefore, children delivered via C-section are deficient in certain "good" bacteria, which explains why these children are at greater risk for allergies, asthma, diabetes, etc. Soon (even within hours), family, friends, nurses, etc., begin to add their flora to the baby.

Thus, not surprisingly, populations of bacteria in humans are more similar among family members than among strangers, probably due to their common diets and bacterial environment.

(2)   Functions of Our Symbiotic Intestinal Bacteria

As stated above, our gut bacteria are in symbiotic relationships with us and each other. As outlined in table 6.3, our intestinal bacteria digest cellulose, proteins, sugars, and lipids, which our intestinal cells cannot do. Studies in animals have shown that approximately 30% of the foods/calories a mammal eats are processed by the gut bacteria which, in turn, secrete the processed nutrients for their intestinal cells to absorb. This is suspected to occur in humans as well. In return, the bacteria receive protection, free housing, food, and for some species, the needed anaerobic conditions. Our intestinal bacteria also manufacture and secrete vitamins such as vitamins K, B_2, B_5, B_7, B_9, B_{12}, and C, which our intestinal cells absorb and our bodies require from food. Normally, our good gut bacteria out-compete pathogens and parasites, and even produce antibacterial toxins to keep the bad bacteria from flourishing in order to protect themselves and ultimately us. We have intestinal disorders, either temporary or long-term, when the good gut bacteria fail to compete.

As shown by Yasunenko et al (2012) at the Washington University, St. Louis, and others, similar to our skin bacteria, each person has a unique population of intestinal bacteria. This population is determined not so much by our genetic makeup, rather by our diets, and our environment (family, housing, neighborhood, work, etc.). Even identical twins differ in their gut microbiomes as much as other siblings or non-relatives, especially if their diet is different. This

Table 6.3

Bacteria in Human GI Tract
(124 European adults)

Total No. Bacteria/Human:	100 Trillion (100 x 10^{12})
	(10X no. of human cells)
Total number species identified in124 people:	>1000
Total number of species worldwide:	~ 5000 – 35,000
Total bacterial genes/all humans:	~3.3 Million (3.3 x 10^6)
	(1000X total genes in human body)
Total number of identified species/human:	~500 (~100 species common in all)
Bacterial genes per each human:	~536,112

Functions of Bacterial Genes
- Adherence to host cells
- Harvesting sugars,
   eg. pectins and sorbitols from plants
- Vitamin production
- Reproduction
- Hormone (neurotransmitters) production

Disease Correlations – Unique Bacterial Populations are found in:
- Obese vs non obese
- Diabetic vs non diabetic
- Healthy vs Crohn's vs Irritable bowel

Comparative Microbiotics in Human Intestine:
- The microbiomes between identical twins are as different
   as those between other siblings
- Diet and environment play a bigger role in determining
   the microbiome than genetics or gender
- The more different the ethnic environment, the more
   different the microbiomes

Data taken from Gerwitz et al, 2010; Qin et al, 2010; Yatsunenko et al, 2012
(Thomas C. Spelsberg, 2012)

difference is greater when siblings, including twins, live separately and eat more diversely. These bacterial populations remain fairly stable in each of us when we maintain unchanged diets or environment where we live. Interestingly, our appendix, originally thought to be a discarded remnant, is now thought to be a reservoir of our natural healthy gut bacteria, and thus, helps maintain or replenish the intestinal population upon demand. The microbial communities in our intestines resemble those secreted in our feces. One gram of our feces contains trillions of live and dead bacteria. These bacteria have been entrapped and discarded along with our own dead intestinal cells and viruses. In fact, bacteria make up 40–60% of the dry weight of human feces. One class of anaerobic bacteria, called methanogens of the archea branch, produce methane and sulfur derived from protein breakdown, to generate our intestinal gas (flatulence). Today, popular "over the counter," probiotic medicines containing good bacteria, are available to help our good gut bacteria remain in control and subdue bad bacteria. This is the goal and popularity of probiotic products sold in stores. These pre- and probiotics often help us when consumed properly.

(3)   Benefits of Human Breast Milk

Breast milk generates the best gut flora (e.g., *Bifidobacterium*) in infants to keep pathogens (i.e., bad bacteria) at bay. Thus, nursing (mother's milk) provides much needed good bacteria to infants, much more than bottle-fed dairy milk or formula. Recent studies by Shugart, Bode, and colleagues, of the University of California-San Diego and Davis, have identified that specific sugars in human breast milk play a major role in maintaining good gut bacteria in humans, e.g., *Bifidobacterium*. These sugars are not found in cow's milk. These sugars have evolved over millions of years of evolution of primates and today protect human infants. The sugars are eaten by bad bacteria as a decoy sugar nutrient, causing them to weaken and die. There are now start-up companies producing these small sugars in the laboratories for treating babies with intestinal disorders.

(4)   Summary of the Digestive Tract Microbes

Our intestinal microbiome can be viewed as an independent organ. Originally acquired at birth (via the birth canal and contact with people around us), the microbiome helps steer our development, immune system, brain functions (discussed later), and metabolic pathways for energy storage and consumption. They perform vital functions: digesting food, extracting crucial elements and minerals, and protecting us against pathogenic (disease-causing) bacterial infections. They regulate our immune system to be accepted as a co-host and thus reduce inflammation. In the womb our intestines are bacteria free, but during passage through the birth canal, we gain our first wave of bacteria on our skin, in our mouths, and in our intestines. This population is further altered by bacteria added by nurses and other family members and even pets, bed sheets, pillows, blankets, etc. All in all, the intestines of babies and adults end up with thousands of species of bacteria with each person having a total of 3.3 million bacterial genes (150 times that of the human genome).

As stated above, many of these genes provide needed functions that humans do not have (see table 6.4). Examples include bacterial production of vitamins and the digestion of foods such as complex carbohydrates (sugars) from plant foods, including apples, potatoes, wheat, and oranges. Many of these bacterial digested products are then absorbed by our intestines. In a way, humans are not that different from cows or other ruminants, in that both use their stomach bacteria to help digest foods. Scientists now know that there are other benefits of our microbiome.

E.   Our Symbiotic Gut Bacteria Maintain Our Health and Disposition

(1)   Overview

Humans have had the erroneous belief that all bacteria are bad for us. Now we know that a multitude of good bacteria, living in symbiosis with us, are helping with food digestion and fighting bad bacteria, producing vitamins, assisting our immune system, and even affecting our mental state (see table 6.4 for a full list of most of these helpful functions). Recent studies have indicated that intestinal flora can malfunction, causing or encouraging Crohn's disease, colitis, irritable bowel syndrome, obesity, diabetes, heart disease, intestinal inflammation, rheumatoid arthritis, multiple sclerosis, and even autism. This malfunction is termed "dysbiosis." Not surprisingly, populations of microbes in the gut are generally specific to people with these diseases or those with certain metabolic syndromes, such as obesity.

Scientists from several institutions have reported that the microbes from obese versus non-obese mice were different. Recent studies have even shown that lean and obese human twins have different intestinal bacteria. The transplanting of the gut bacteria of the lean twin into the gut of the obese twin causes the latter to lose weight. When non-obese mice were given the bacteria from obese mice, they ate excessively and gained weight. They even acquired the obese mouse's hunger neurohormone patterns. The stomach produces these hormones that regulate the brain centers to signal the feeling of hunger. The reverse pattern of neurohormones occurred when obese mice were given bacteria

Table 6.4

Helpful Functions of Intestinal Bacteria in Humans

- Breaks down complex carbohydrates

- Produces Vitamins B-2, B-5, B-7, B-9, B-12, and C, thymine, and riboflavin

- Breaks down intestinal mucin protein

- Absorbs and processes simple sugars

- Generates iron for hemoglobin

- Generates appetite suppressing PYY hormone

- Regulate fat deposits in humans generating fatty acids

- Affects energy conversion in muscles and liver by generating chemical signals

- Produces polysaccharide A (PSA) that binds to dendritic cells that cause T cells to produce interleukin to reduce inflammation

- Influences the immune system development and inflammation

- Produces hormones and neurotransmitters that affect the brain and mental state

- Regulates our mental disposition (moods), hunger, obesity, and mental disorders

(Thomas C. Spelsberg, 2012)

from non-obese mice. Frazier, and colleagues, at the University of Maryland, recently identified the species of gut bacteria in humans, which were specifically associated with a good (lean) or a bad (obese) metabolic state. This topic is further discussed later in this chapter.

It has recently been established that when we are young, our gut bacteria help to develop our immune system, including the stimulation of the immune system to make antibodies against the bad pathogens. Young children raised with a lot of bacterial exposure, such as on farms, or having pets such as dogs, have immune systems regulated for optimal immune function and disease resistance. As adults, these exposed children have less intestinal diseases, asthma, rheumatoid arthritis, and other autoimmune diseases, than do city-raised children. This protection lasts for one's lifetime. A specific strain of bacteria, *Lactobacillus johnsonii*, has been identified by Lynch and coworkers at the University of California, San Francisco, as the primary source of the protection provided by animals against allergies and asthma in humans. This bacterial strain obviously provides substances that stimulate our early immune system.

Recent studies at Harvard University and elsewhere have shown that the degree of general immune based inflammation and related bowel diseases are increased in lab animals raised in sterile conditions. The immune system operated better (more normal) when the animals were born and raised in a natural, non-sterile, and bacterial laden, environment. These results might explain why human youth, raised on farms, are healthier (less allergies) than those raised in a city. We can conclude that the early exposure to a variety of bacteria (good and bad) probably creates a more powerful immune system with conditioned immune stem cells that are better prepared to respond quickly and more efficiently to exposures later in life.

In summary, our normal symbiotic gut bacteria help keep us healthy. Our bodies become ill with intestinal diseases when these good bacterial populations diminish and are replaced with bad (pathogenic or disease-causing) populations. Table 6.5 lists various diseases in humans caused by different species of pathogenic bacteria. The incidence of other diseases such as cancer, diabetes, asthma, metabolic syndrome, and obesity, appear to increase when our microbiome is disturbed. The bacteria around us can also affect our health. For example, house dust causes allergies in many people. The cause of much of this allergic response has been found to be the proteins of dead bacteria in our environment. Specific effects of a disturbed microbiome on various human diseases are discussed below.

(2)   <u>Some Specifics on Intestinal Inflammation/Ulcers/Colitis: There is Power in Our Poop</u>

Recent studies of lab animals, raised in sterile conditions and thus have no gut bacteria, have demonstrated an underdeveloped immune system. One species of our gut bacteria, *bacteriodes fragilis* (*B fragilis*), lives in 70 to 80% of people, and produces polysaccharide A (PSA), which maintains a healthy intestine and a balance between our immune system and the microbes in our intestines. Lab animals without this bacteria developed colitis. The PSA activates the immune regulatory cells that aid in developing our immune system and dampens the inflammation caused by the pro-inflammatory T cells. Unfortunately, scientists in the United States are now finding that average humans are beginning to lose their

Table 6.5

Diseases Caused or Encouraged by Pathogenic Bacteria

Bacterial Species	Infections/Diseases
Staphylococcus	infections, gangrene, sepsis
Streptococcus	Gangrene, sepsis, strep throat, skin infections, flesh eating infections, pneumonia
Clostridium	gangrene, tetanus, botulism
Mycoplasma	respiratory infections
Rickettsiae	Rocky Mountain spotted fever
Yersinia Pesti	bubonic plague
Haemophilisis	meningitis, deafness, pneumonia, sinusitis, bronchitis
Bordetella	whooping cough
C. Diphtheria	diphtheria
Legionnella	Legionnaire's disease
Mycobacterium	tuberculosis, leprosy
Chlamydia	pelvic inflammation
Treponema	syphilis
Prevotella copri	autoimmune diseases, rheumatoid arthritis

(Thomas C. Spelsberg, 2013)

intestinal *B fragilis*, therefore causing the current increase in the frequency of inflammatory/autoimmune diseases, obesity, and other immune disorders, in our population. Another bacterium, *H. pylori*, modulates the acidic conditions produced by the stomach and calms the stomach. If too much acid is produced, they secrete substances to neutralize the acid. What is not fully understood is how *H. pylori* can also cause/enhance stomach ulcers. One speculation is that other substances, produced by *H. pylori*, may encourage stomach ulcers when overproduced. Maybe these bacteria cause this by simply invading our tissues via "leaky guts" created by inflammation. When inflammation occurs in the gut, *H. pylori* and other bacteria invade the intestinal lining and even enter our blood stream and cause ulcers via the "leaky gut" situation. Stomach ulcers are now treated with antibiotics with marked success.

As gross as it seems, physicians are beginning to use enriched intestinal bacteria from feces of family members to treat other family members with bowel disorders and obesity. Believe it or not, this approach seems to be working. This procedure is called "fecal microbiota transplant." Table 6.6 outlines the current approaches in this field. A pioneer in fecal transplants is Dr. Thomas Brody of Australia. He has successfully used this technique to treat thousands of patients with colitis and irritable bowel and Crohn's disease. Dr. Kelly, Providence, RI, and Dr. Brandt, Montefiore Medical Center in New York, have also transplanted fecal bacteria from healthy family members to many sick family members with excellent results in curing or calming bowel disorders. Similar studies are now being conducted by Drs. Orenstein, DiBaise, Khanna, and Pardi, at the Mayo Clinic in the United States, as well as by other scientists in Europe. I guess we can now state that there is "Power in our Poop".

Table 6.6

Correcting GI Disorders Using Fecal Bacteria

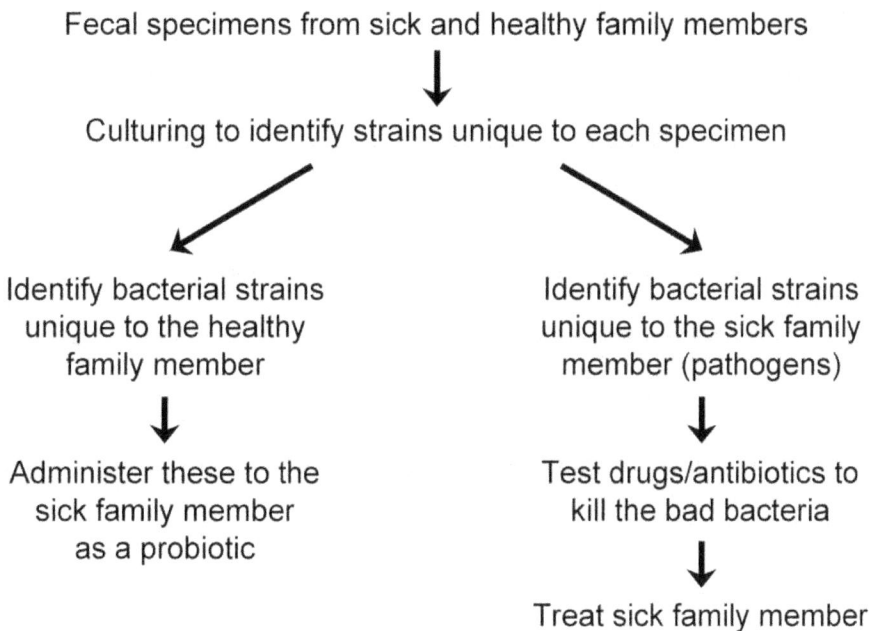

Fecal specimens from sick and healthy family members

↓

Culturing to identify strains unique to each specimen

Identify bacterial strains unique to the healthy family member	Identify bacterial strains unique to the sick family member (pathogens)
↓	↓
Administer these to the sick family member as a probiotic	Test drugs/antibiotics to kill the bad bacteria
	↓
	Treat sick family member

(Thomas C. Spelsberg, 2013)

(3)   Intestinal Microbes and Our Immune System

Scientists are gaining knowledge on how the trillions of bacteria in our intestines and on our skin communicate with our immune system. Recent studies have revealed that the whole immune system is affected by the bacteria in our intestines. When encountering pathogens which have invaded our intestinal lining and blood, the pro-inflammatory T cells, which fight infection, release toxic compounds to destroy infectious pathogens. However, these toxins hurt our own tissues, encouraging inflammatory and autoimmune diseases such as colitis, Crohn's disease, type I diabetes, and multiple sclerosis. Studies by Mazmanian and co-workers at the California Institute of Technology have demonstrated that the early exposure of certain good bacteria to newborns and children, help prepare their immune system to better deal with bad pathogenic microbes later in life. This early exposure better regulates T cell secretion of toxins to destroy the pathogens or better prepares the immune stem cells to recognize and accept such pathogens. All of the above has added to the earlier described concept: being raised in a sterile environment is harmful to your health, and has a negative impact on your health throughout your lifetime. It is now accepted that the early exposure of our immune system to the microbial world helps to develop a more effective and efficient immune system. It is now believed that our immune system's long-term memory T cells are responsible for these long-term memory responses in our guts.

(4)   Stomach Hunger Hormone/Obesity/Diabetes

Recent studies in lab animals have shown that the stomach bacteria, H. pylori, also regulate the neuro-hormone, ghrelin,that is produced by the cells of our stomach and intestines. Ghrelin tells the brain that you are hungry. After you eat, ghrelin levels drop, and you feel satisfied with no need to eat. Without *H. pylori* in their stomachs, the animals became obese because the ghrelin levels did not decrease and the animals continued eating. When these bacteria were returned to the stomachs of these animals, the ghrelin levels returned to normal patterns, decreasing after a meal and telling the animals to stop eating. It is speculated that the bacteria produce a substance which regulates the ghrelin production by the stomach cells. This phenomenon is called "Interkingdom Signaling." Humans also produce and use ghrelin for the same purpose. Interestingly, 80% of Americans living 60 years ago, hosted *H. pylori*, and overall were much thinner. Today only 6% of Americans have H. pylori in adequate amounts, and most individuals without *H. pylori* are significantly overweight with the consequences of a much higher frequency of diabetes. Thus, we have new generations of people without *H. pylori* and no regulation of ghrelin, with the resulting epidemic of obesity. Some scientists feel it is the constant barrage of antibiotics that has encouraged this "epidemic" loss of *H. pylori* bacteria along with ghrelin/appetite regulation, and it is probably part of the cause of obesity in the world's human populations.

Differences in the microbial populations have now been found in lean versus obese humans, and in certain families but not others. The populations of bacteria associated with obesity in humans are also less diverse (which is unhealthy) and display an emphasis on sugar, lipid, and amino acid metabolism. The human and animal gut bacteria population seems to reflect an energy balance including the efficiency of calories harvested from foods. The particular species of bacteria in the population are determined by the diet and the species which, in turn, determine the efficiency of calories harvested. Even a person's last meal plays a role in the rapid growth (and death) of bacteria. New studies have revealed that firmicute bacteria are associated with (and may encourage) obesity, while the

B fragilis bacteria (like *H. pylori* discussed above) inhibits obesity and encourages leanness. One species, *A. kermansia muciniphila*, also seems to help prevent obesity and diabetes in mice. Overall, these results indicate that some bacteria produce substances which encourage leanness, while others produce substances that encourage obesity or cause intestinal disease.

Studies reported in 2013 by Patterson, Gonzalez, and Mitchell, at the NIH/NCI, suggest that the diet may also regulate the levels of *Lactobacillus*. This can result in the decrease in bile acid which inhibits the farnesoid X receptor which, in turn, regulates sugar and fats in the body. Further, some "bad" bacteria produce high amounts of cholesterol and lipids, which are absorbed and enhance inflammation and obesity, both of which are bad for the heart and vessels. Other bad bacterial species produce selective sugars which over-stimulate the immune system and encourage inflammation in the bowels and disease. Recent studies, published by Markle et al, have shown that bacteria in the intestines of non-obese mice also regulate sex hormone production and minimize inflammation caused by autoimmunity. The latter also helps prevent the development of diabetes and a metabolic syndrome. Similarly, Smith et al (2013), have identified bacteria-produced fatty acids which regulate our regulatory T cells and immune system. Overall, the human microbiome plays a role in our overall health, the states of our immune system and inflammation, and our propensity for a metabolic syndrome.

(5)   Our Gut Bacteria Control How We Feel and Behave (Including Autistic Symptoms)

Our gut bacteria, which are unique to each of us, regulate not only our health, our immune system, but also appear to play a role in our stress levels, anxiety, and depression. In short, our gut bacteria have many influences on our general mental well being and mood. Dr. Patterson and colleagues at the California Institute of Technology, and Drs. David and Turnbaugh, and colleagues at Harvard University, reported that populations of gut bacteria can change in one day with changing diet. Certain gut bacteria produce factors which are injected directly into the intestinal cells to affect signaling pathways. Recently, some of these bacterial factors have been shown to influence our behavior by producing precursors to serotonin, noradrenaline, dopamine, and neurotransmitters. In addition to the ghrelin-hunger-bacteria pathway discussed above, scientists have recently identified a novel microbiome-gut-brain axis with evidence that the species of bacteria in our intestines have an affect on the vagus nerve. This results in mood/emotional control, as well as brain activities and functions, such as memory. Interestingly, certain species of bacteria can enhance or decrease the symptoms of autism in animal models. Reductions in *B fragilis* caused increased autistic symptoms. A chemical in the blood, 4-ethylphenylsulfate (similar to para-cresol in humans), increased when *B fragilis* decreased, and was shown to cause the autistic symptoms. Other recent studies have revealed that bacteria found in lean people produce greater amounts of substances which help us sleep and build/repair brain tissue. These results explain why the proper use of probiotics (good bacteria) and healthy diets have often shown favorable outcomes to improve one's mood and health.

F.   The Body's Natural Defenses against Invading "Bad/Toxic" Bacteria

As discussed above, exposure of young children to a variety of (good) bacteria early in their life, fine-tunes the immune system to respond properly and efficiently to acute and low grade infections. It also prevents chronic inflammation later in life. The opposite happens if a lack of bacterial exposure occurs. The latter encourages heart attacks, strokes, diabetes, cancer, and autoimmune diseases later in life. Of the thousands of bacteria species in each human, only about 100 species of bacteria are known to be pathogenic (disease-causing). All humans harbor some of these bad bacteria (table 6.1), but most of us remain healthy due to our body's natural defenses, including the presence of good bacteria, our immune system, and our individual cells' own defense mechanisms. However, the "bad" bacteria are opportunists and will "attack and take over" when our body's defense weakens or when the bad bacteria develop new strategies. Table 6.1 lists the 3 most prominent "pathogenic bacteria" which are harbored by most humans: table 6.5 lists diseases these and others cause in humans. *Mycobacteria* which cause tuberculosis and leprosy are harbored in 33% of people in the world, while 50% of people in the world are estimated to harbor *H. pylori* which can cause stomach ulcers and stomach cancers, and 50% of us harbor *Staphylococcus aureus*, which can cause staph infections on the skin and in the respiratory system. Infectious diseases caused by bacteria, viruses, or parasites, are the second leading cause of deaths worldwide, behind heart, but ahead of cancer and other organ failures. The battle between the good and bad bacteria is always ongoing - morning, noon, and night.

(1)   The Strategies of Bad (Pathogenic) Bacteria: Negative Effects over a Lifetime

Pathogenic bacteria are often subversive in their actions. Some will attach to our cells and alter our cell's metabolism and functions to fit their needs, so they can multiply. They often secrete toxins to subdue the neighboring good bacteria as well as our cells, resulting in illnesses.

Here is a list of the strategies that some pathogenic bacteria use to survive:

1)   secrete factors that prevent themselves from being eaten by our macrophages

2)   secrete toxins to alter or kill human intestinal cells. Examples of such toxins are diphtheria toxin, cholera toxin, anthrax toxin, pertussis toxins, tetanus toxin, and botulism toxin

3)   alter recognition sites on their membranes to avoid detection by the immune system and good bacteria

4)   secrete degrading enzymes to destroy our tissues

5)   secrete growth factors and adhesives to help themselves grow, form plagues/biofilms, and enhance blood flow to themselves to gain nourishment and allow their toxins to travel to other parts of the body

6)   attach themselves to active, biologically important "receptors" on the membranes of our own cells to disrupt the cells' natural signaling/ communication network, after which they "take control" of the cell

7)   inject effector /reprogramming agents directly into our cells to plunder nutrients and to reprogram our cells to do their bidding; and finally

8)   encourage their own engulfment by host (human) cells so that they can reprogram them as an insider.

This reprogramming of our human cells, as well as eliminating our good bacteria, are the primary causes of inflammation, resulting in more deaths of neighboring good bacteria and allowing the bad bacteria to propagate (survive). Examples of the diseases and intestinal pathogenic bacteria which use the above tactics are outlined in table 6.5 and include tuberculosis, Legionnaires' disease,

Crohn's disease, bubonic plague, and salmonella poisoning. Their infections cause dysentery, vomiting, fever, organ failure, cancer, and sometimes death.

Interestingly, recent studies have indicated that pathogenic (bacterial) infections often don't end when the "illness" is apparently over. There is evidence for lifelong consequences. The Center for Disease Control and Prevention (CDCP) estimates in 2011 in the United States alone, there were 48 million illnesses (vomiting, diarrhea, etc.),128,000 hospitalizations, and 3000 deaths due to ingested pathogenic bacterial organisms. The cost to the economy was $6.7 billion. Now, scientists at the CDCP have evidence that some of these sick people (approximately 10 to 20%) later report long-term chronic symptoms suspected to be a result of these diseases, e.g., hypertension, reactive arthritis, renal impairment, ulcerative colitis, aortic aneurysms, and joint/muscle pain. These body responses due to these lingering bacterial illnesses can last from years to a lifetime. One wonders whether this is caused by lingering (hiding) pathogenic bacteria in the chronically ill patients.

(2)   Our Bodies' Defense Strategy against the Pathogenic Bacteria

To combat the above, our bodies have developed amazing defenses against bacteria and viruses. Our cells have evolved defense mechanisms with both internal and external alarms to defend themselves. Our cells defend against these pathogenic bacteria by instigating extracellular inflammation to alarm our immune system. Many of our cells do this even as they are dying in the fight. Many of our inflammatory/immune cells have membrane receptors (called "toll" receptors) that recognize many bacteria membrane proteins and attack the bacteria. Our macrophages engulf the bad bacteria into their internal cell "inflamasomes" that destroys the bacteria. When all else fails, some of our cells will even commit suicide (apoptosis) to help destroy the bad bacteria for the good of the whole. This more powerful, last line of defense by our macrophages, has recently been shown to involve the promotion of programmed cell death, called pyroptosis. This process is activated by certain strong pathogens which cause tuberculosis and other diseases. The human cell, when losing the battle to bad bacteria, will secrete suicide inflammatory signals (cytokines) to encourage macrophages and dendritic cells to attack and devour host (human) cells, including the bad bacteria, in the neighborhood. These dead cells often trap the bad bacteria for body excretion into feces. Sadly, these inflammatory signals also create extreme inflammatory responses causing damage to good tissues.

Recent studies have revealed other mechanisms used by our cells to protect us and destroy bad bacteria and other pathogens (fungi, mold, etc.). For example, our intestinal cells produce small proteins, "alpha defensins," which form "extracellular" meshes to physically block bacterial invasions into our gut cells. These proteins also can directly kill a variety of bacteria and viruses. As outlined in table 6.7, a potent mechanism of defense by our immune cells involves their production of chemicals, called mono- and di-chlorotaurine, that kill bacteria, fungi, protozoa, and even viruses inside our macrophages once these organisms have been engulfed by the immune cells (white blood cells/macrophages). These substances act within minutes to destroy the pathogens, while having very low toxicity to our own cells. These substances are being examined as possible antimicrobial therapeutic drugs, especially since pathogens have never generated resistance to these particular chemicals. It should be reminded that a negative

Table 6.7

A Novel Combatant to Antimicrobial Therapy, Including Drug Resistance, Using Our Own Cells Defense Chemical

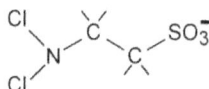

$$\begin{array}{c} Cl \\ | \\ Cl \end{array} N - \overset{|}{\underset{|}{C}} - \overset{|}{\underset{|}{C}} - SO_3^-$$

1. Mono- and Di-chlorotaurine is used by our own white blood cells to kill bacteria, fungi, protozoa, and viruses once they are engulfed into the cells.
2. Acts in minutes while antibiotics need hours.
3. No host resistance ever occurs.
4. Very lethal to drug/antibiotic resistant microbes.
5. Very low toxicity to our cells but a potent, rapidly acting lethal agent to cell microbes.
6. 500X less toxic on normal (host) cells and kills within minutes (not hours as for antibiotics).
7. Lethal to drug resistant bacteria and fungi and blocks viral spread in hosts.
8. Penetrates all areas, even where antibiotics do not.

Information taken from Low et al 2009, Bioorganic and Medicinal Chem Letters 19, 196-198.
Francovilla et al 2009, Bioorganic and Medicinal Chem Letters 19, 2731-2734.
Weiss et al 1982, J. Clin Invest 70, 598-607.

outcome of the inflammatory defense is that extensive inflammation can lead to damage of good tissues and organs resulting in long-term secondary diseases such as heart disease, Alzheimer's, cancer, and diabetes.

(3)　　How Bacteria become Resistant to Vaccines, Antibiotics, and our Immune System

As counter attacks, bad bacterial and viral pathogens are constantly devising techniques to avoid both our immune system (e.g., bubonic plague, Legionnaire's disease, AIDS, and hepatitis), and some of the internal defenses of our cells (e.g., dysentery, hepatitis, tuberculosis, and some cases of Crohn's disease). These pathogenic bacteria struggle to survive as all living entities do. There are numerous articles in journals and books on the mechanisms of antibiotic resistance in bacteria. Antibiotic resistance is a big problem worldwide, especially in hospitals and schools, and is hampered by the lack of knowledge of the mechanisms of how many antibiotics work. The mechanisms of these resistances involve:

1)　　preventing the entrance of the antibiotic into the bacterial cell

2)　　inactivation of the antibiotic via binding to large molecules inside the bacteria

3)　　direct destruction or inactivation of the antibiotic by enzyme proteins

4)　　use of large mucoid colonies which prevent the immune system's macrophages from engulfing these bacteria.

Interestingly, most antimicrobial resistance, whatever the mechanism, is encoded by mobile genetic elements. For example, the ability to form mucoid colonies has been found to be due to the activation of a gene, yrfFA, by the local insertion of a transposon. The latter permits the relative easy horizontal gene transfer of resistance even between different species of bacteria, and thus, encourages the spread of resistance among a population. Further, it only takes one bacteria out of millions to gain this attribute. This one cell then begins to divide, replacing the dead bacteria, ending up predominating by selective advantage, as a population of millions in a few days. These resistant cells also cause neighboring bacteria to become resistant by horizontal gene transfer using infectious transposons with the attached resistance genes.

In addition, an effective strategy by pathogenic bacteria and a major problem for humans is that, under stress (e.g., when exposed to antibiotics), many bacterial species shut down (become dormant), forming inactive spores protected against almost all threats. They will then reawaken when the threat is removed. Recent studies have shown that when a bacterial population (bad or good bacteria) is threatened, 25% of the bacterial cells will shut down (i.e., will have no growth or cell division), thereby becoming resistant to antibiotics and extremes in the environment. In this stage, they are also able to incorporate DNA (genes) from the environment, including neighboring viruses and transposons from other bacteria into their own cells, again using "horizontal gene transfer." This feat significantly expands their genomes and their capabilities for survival, including antibiotic resistance.

Thus, both the bad and good bacteria quickly adapt to various environmental, chemical, and antibiotic challenges to become resistant to any threats to their survival. It is a constant ongoing war. By acquiring external bacterial genes (transferred) from other bacteria, and through the use of genetic adaptation via possible epigenetic mechanisms (gene regulation) within their own gene pool, most bacteria populations eventually become resistant to most threats/therapies.

This is life's plan to help all living entities to adapt and survive. It is interesting to note that scientists have found that approximately 80% of "acquired" new genes in bacteria come from other neighboring bacteria via direct exchange of genes (horizontal gene transfer) by transposons or by the invasion of viruses, carrying resistant genes with them. Scientists are devising new drugs to attach and defeat these known resistance pathways of defense to help cure these diseases and infections. Much is still unknown. The battle continues on and thus, our body's inner war on disease has always been and probably will always be present, mainly due to the adaptability of the bacteria. It should be reminded that all life forms on Earth will interact with each other if they share the same space/environment. They will compete as well as cooperate with each other for food, health, and survival, and even share their genes.

G.   Bacteria on Our Money: More Roots of Evil

As we all know, money is a necessary tool of human societies, but it is also the root of much evil in our world. People live for it, love for it, steal for it, deceive for it, give birth for it, and even kill for it. It is the basis of greed and insecurities. A hidden evil of money (especially paper money) is its contamination with drugs (narcotics), and bad "bacteria." Paper money not only harbors a multitude of good bacteria but also a multitude of bad bacteria; 3000 species in all. These bacteria often end up on our hands and then on the things we touch, including our eyes, nose, and our mouths. Recent analysis of hundreds of bills and coins showed millions of bacteria on both paper money and coins, including human fecal bacteria. Interestingly, 90% of the bills from in the big cities contained traces of the drug cocaine, which is much more stable than heroin, and obviously originated from the drug industry.

H.   Human Viruses and Disease

It should be mentioned that infectious viruses reside in humans and all animals and plants, and are even more abundant than bacteria. There are an estimated 10^{31} viruses on Earth and 10^{16} (100 x million x billion) viruses in each human. Viruses are simple organisms, 100 times smaller than bacteria and are comprised of DNA or RNA surrounded by a protein coat. Overall, most viruses are destroyed by the acid in the stomach or by being trapped and discarded along with our dying/dead bacterial and intestinal cells. They are also absorbed or destroyed by our immune system or by our good bacteria that they invade. Viruses survive by invading the bacterial cells in our intestines, as well as our gut cells using specific receptors on the larger target (host) cell. They may reside there quietly for a while but the ultimate goal is to redirect our cells' and our gut microbes' replication machinery and nutrient production for their own survival.

Viruses are infectious and opportunistic. Viruses often spend most of their lives hidden within animal and plant cells and bacteria. On the good side (for us) viruses assist in the exchange of genes between bacteria, plant, and animal cells, allowing bacteria (and themselves) to rapidly adapt to new challenges and survive. On the bad side, infectious viruses replicate themselves, with some rupturing the host cells, often making cells sick (diseased), or even killing them and releasing still more viruses to infect additional healthy cells. As a defense against viral infections, our cells often block the ability of invading viruses to replicate themselves by destroying the viral genetic material. Alternatively, our virally induced sick cells send signals to our immune system that destroy our diseased cells along with the viruses. Using genomic DNA analyses, human feces have been shown to contain over 1000 different types of viruses, which obviously have invaded our gut bacteria and our gut cells to ultimately be defecated along with the gut bacteria and human intestinal cells.

It is interesting to note that there are 100 viruses for every bacteria in us (Pennisi, E., 2011). That calculates to approximately 10^{16} (or 10 quadrillion) viruses in the intestinal flora of every human body. In fact, in every gram of human stool, there are 10 billion (10^{10}) dead/inactivated or active viruses. It has been found that sick children (with fever) have 10 times the amount of viruses in their blood than children without fever. Thus, like bacteria, viruses are opportunistic, replicating and attacking when the host is sick, with the sole purpose to survive and reproduce as much as they can, especially when our defenses are weak. The global population of the common cold virus among all humans has been estimated to exceed 10^{21} virions (1 billion x trillion). They have been very successful in surviving throughout eternity.

Ancient viral genomes have been found buried in human DNA with most classified as transposons and retrotransposons (jumping genes). As described in Chapter 7, these can make up over 50% of our genome due to self-duplication. These appear to have originated from ancient viral infections of pre-human ancestors, and adopted by our cells for useful functions. Some are estimated to be as old as 93 million years – much older than many primates and the human species. Some viruses probably have no effect on humans, some may help us, but many hurt us. Some may act through our microbiome. Remember, there are 100 viruses in our bodies for every bacteria, some residing in our cells but most residing in our bacteria. It is amazing that there are approximately 10^{16} viruses in each of us.

I.   Conclusions and Current Progress

Our symbiotic microbiome represents a population 10 times that of our own cells. Our skin bacteria and mouth bacteria can protect or harm us. Bacteria can protect or cause tooth decay, skin infections, and internal inflammations, depending on the species. In any event, one can now say to friends and colleagues, "Lets shake hands, exchange our bacteria, and agree" or "Lets kiss, exchange bacteria, and make up."

The population of an individual's gut (intestinal) microbiome dictates the disposition towards a variety of inflammatory diseases and metabolic states (e.g., obesity), as well as mental disorders. The gut microbiome affects brain functions and influences brain chemistry, behavior, anxiety, stress, and depression. This is achieved mainly by affecting the vagus nerve and altering our hunger. Some scientists have claimed bacteria have a bigger impact on what enters our blood stream than our own eating habits. Interestingly, scientists are changing rodent behaviors, disposition, eating habits, and disease incidence by changing their gut bacteria. Scientists are now giving people with colitis and irritable bowels the bacteria from feces of healthy family members which displace the bad bacteria and are observing marked success in eliminating the disease symptoms.

The human intestinal microbiome population is a major factor in the regulation of obesity. To accomplish these feats, our gut bacteria secrete factors and nutrients to be absorbed by our own gut cells. Through this chemical signaling, our gut microbes regulate our intestinal lining cells, and alter the production of intestinal hormones (e.g., ghrelin and leptin), which in turn, signal the brain as to hunger or satiety (full stomach). Not unexpected, obese people have unique gut microbes compared to lean people, even within the same families, and display

116

abnormal regulation of the hunger hormones, ghrelin and leptin. Lean people and animals have a diverse population of gut bacteria while obese people have a much less diverse bacterial population. Giving lean animals or humans the gut bacteria of obese animals causes the former to modestly gain weight. In contrast, giving obese animals and humans the bacteria from lean animals and humans respectively, causes the obese to markedly lose weight and have less inflammation. It is interesting to note that the United States Agency for International Development (USAID) has estimated that by 2005, the world's adult human population weighed approximately 287 million tons (i.e., 574 billion pounds or 5.7×10^{11} pounds). About 15 million tons is due to obesity involving 500 million people. The United States alone makes up one-third of the world's human obesity problem. Humans need to change their gut microbes. Bad bacteria cause inflammation and play a role in enhancing one's metabolic syndrome. As described above, scientists now believe that altering our gut microbes will (and does) alter the bacterial effects on our metabolism, including obesity, and improve our metabolic syndrome level, and our disposition.

Finally, it should be reminded that certain powerful antibiotics are derived from good bacteria which they used to combat enemy bacteria. For example, streptomycin, erythromycin, and tetracyclines are produced by and obtained from *Streptomyces* bacteria. Bacitrins and polymyxin are isolated from *Bacillus* bacteria and so on. There may be value in using "probiotics," including yogurt, that provides "good" bacteria for our guts. However, the fecal transplants seem to have the most effect and success. In any case, our good gut microbes act as typical symbiotes: processing food and providing vitamins, while receiving food and protection, and determining our own health. Recent studies have shown that certain gut microbes can inactivate drugs that may explain why some individuals do not respond to certain drugs.

Scientists are now profiling the gut bacteria in people with intestinal disorders in order to prevent or cure diseases, including intestinal cancer. Recently, scientists at the Genome Institute in Singapore, reported that Helicobacter Pylori induced mutations in the DNA of eukaryote cells in culture, many in cancer related genes, causing the cells to transform into cancer cells. The DNA repair processes in the Eukaryote cells is blocked, thereby enhancing the DNA damage. In 2013, the pharmaceutical giant, Johnson & Johnson, established a $6.5 million deal with Second Genome, a microbiome start-up company, to develop treatments to alter the gut microbiome population to treat/cure patients with intestinal diseases. Recent publications in *Nature Communications* (2013) from Penn State University and the National Cancer Institute by Drs. Patterson, Gonzalez, and Mitchell, reported that giving animals a strong antioxidant, Tempol, caused weight reductions by altering the intestinal microbiome. Overall, health and metabolic state were improved with this drug. Novel antioxidant drugs may be derived from these studies to induce weight loss. In any event, we are fortunate that we are aware of our microbiome and the harm or protection from diseases it can bring us. This knowledge emphasizes the fact that our life style will affect our microbiome which, in turn, will affect our metabolic and mental health. This knowledge has and will help in our fight against diseases and obesity.

Section III

The Human Genome and Individualized Medicine

Chapter 7

The Human Genome: Our Genes Determine Who We Are

<u>Definitions</u>

<u>adult stem cells (multipotent)</u>: stem cells in adult tissues that are able to differentiate several adult cell types.

<u>base/nucleotide</u>: primary component of DNA or RNA containing a pyrimidine or purine base attached to a deoxyribose or ribose sugar respectively: one of the genetic triplet code of three bases.

<u>diploid</u>: cells or organisms containing two sets of chromosomes (one maternal set and one paternal set).

<u>epigenome</u>: genes, mostly located in the junk DNA, that code for RNA, but not protein, and regulate the expression of other protein coding genes via epigenetics.

<u>exome</u>: the combined exons of a genome; all domains in a genome that can code for RNA and/or protein.

<u>exon</u>: domains of a gene which are transcriptionally active and code for protein.

<u>exosome (nuclear)</u>: a multi-enzyme complex involved in multiple RNA processing and degradation. Involved in RNA turnover and half-life.

<u>gene</u>: hereditary unit in the genome (DNA in the chromosomes) that codes for functional proteins or RNAs.

<u>genetics</u>: branch of biology concerned with the creation of living species and their heredity.

<u>genomics</u>: field involving the study of the genomes of living creatures.

<u>germ cell</u>: sperm and egg cells of the human body containing only 23 chromosomes and function to join to create an embryo.

haploid: cells or organisms containing one set of chromosomes as found in germ cells, i.e., sperm and egg.

human genome: all the genes (genetic information) carried by a human cell.

intron: domains of a gene which are transcriptionally active (produce RNA) but do not code for protein in the pre-messenger RNA: RNA domains are removed from the pre-messenger RNA before protein production.

junk DNA: an erroneous term formerly applied to the non-functioning parts (90%) of the genome, excluding the protein coding genes. This domain is now known to contain pseudogenes, repetitive DNA, which includes transposons: approximately 75% of the DNA is transcriptionally active (RNA producing but not protein coding) whose genes code for small microRNAs, interfering RNAs, and long non-coding RNAs.

microRNAs, long non-coding RNAs, non-coding RNAs: see Chapter 8.

mitochondria: semi-autonomous self-reproducing cell organelle in eukaryotes that provide energy and oxidation for the cell. These organelles have properties similar to bacteria and may have evolved from them.

non-coding RNA (ncRNA): the term describing all the RNAs which do not code for proteins. These RNAs are transcribed from genes in the "junk DNA" and are involved in epigenetic regulation of the protein coding genes. Examples are the microRNAs and long non-coding RNAs: ribosomal and transfer RNAs are not included.

omics: the total amount of something (Greek): see table 7.6 for list and definitions of various omics.

ontogeny: the complete developmental process of an organism.

repeat sequences: nucleotide sequences that occur repeatedly in the chromosomal DNA (genome): up to 70% of the genome is represented as repetitious sequence families, much of which is created by retrotransposons.

retrotransposons: one kind of transposable elements which replicates itself via RNA intermediates to create extra copies of itself which reinserts elsewhere in the genome; they create repeat sequences; probably originating with viral infections eons ago.

somatic cell: cells of the body containing 46 chromosomes (diploid). See also germ cell.

telomeres: a specialized sequence structure found at the ends of eukaryote chromosomes; structure (domain) contains a small sequence that is repeated up to 60 times but is gradually reduced as cells divide; when shortened, the cells cease to divide and undergo apoptosis; immortal stem cells maintain their telomeres using telemerase enzyme or another unknown mechanism to repair/re-lengthen the telomeres.

transposable elements (also called jumping genes): represented by transposons and retrotransposons. These are mobile DNA elements that can translocate to other locations of the genome and can alter the expression of the protein coding genes thought to have originated from viral genomes. Some replicate themselves to create repeat sequences.

transposons: one of a kind transposable elements which are flanked by repeat sequences. Usually contain functional genes in the middle and often regulate genes neighboring the insertion site.

A. The Human Genome: Properties and Interesting Facts

Most of us have heard about our genes, genetics, chromosomes, and genomics/genomes. This chapter describes their functions, composition, and the information they carry to create each of us.

There is a common genetic link among all life forms, including humans, in that they all use the same basic genetic code in their DNA, the same processes in expressing gene activity, as well as similar gene sequences for coding for proteins and similar functions of these proteins. The term "human genome" refers to all the DNA in a human cell, generally meaning all the DNA in the cell nucleus. This includes all the protein coding and RNA coding genes in all of a human's chromosomes. There is some additional DNA (mitochondrial DNA) in eukaryote organisms, which is discussed later. The suffix "ome" was taken from the Greek language and loosely translated means "mass" or "totality" of something. It was joined with gene to create genome in 1920 by the German scientist, E. M. Winkler. The terms "human genome" and "genomics" (the study of the genome) became popular in the late 1990s and early 2000s, with the achievement of the Human Genome Project. This project involved the DNA sequencing of the entire human genome, i.e., all the DNA in all the chromosomes. Many other scientific fields have adopted the suffix "omics;" this will be discussed at the end of this chapter.

(1) The DNA and Chromosomes

Most cells in the human body have 46 chromosomes, which occur in pairs, one member of each pair originates from the father's sperm and the other member originates from the mother's egg. These cells are classified as diploid cells. The sperm and egg, each with only 23 chromosomes, are classified as haploid. In a diploid cell there is one pair representing the sex chromosomes, which in males, are represented by one X chromosome, donated by the mother, and one Y chromosome, donated by the father. In females, the sex chromosomes are represented by two X chromosomes (one each donated by the father and one from the mother). The remaining 44 chromosomes are called somatic chromosomes. Thus, it is the father's sperm carrying either one Y or one X chromosome that determines the sex of the embryo upon fertilization (i.e., donating an "X" to the egg to generate a female, or a "Y" to generate a male).

Organisms of the same species have chromosomes which have the same size, genetic (gene) organization (gene arrangement), and number of chromosomes. This allows them to properly pair and exchange DNA during sperm/egg production (meiosis) and as well as pair properly during fertilization and subsequent cell divisions (mitosis). The result is a fertilized embryo with a normal diploid set of chromosomes that creates a viable and fertile offspring. Organisms of different species generally have different genetic organization and number of chromosomes and therefore cannot create viable embryos. This is because they cannot form identical chromosome pairs, often resulting in gene losses and failures in germ cell production and/or in development of the organism.

To create a human embryo, and ultimately a baby after fertilization of the sperm and egg, each of the chromosomes, 23 from the sperm and 23 from the egg, join as homologous pairs to create the initial embryonic "somatic" cell with the complete genome of 46 chromosomes required for a living human embryo. Again, this cell represents the fertilized egg and is classified as diploid. This fertilized egg then replicates its DNA (chromosomes) and divides into 2 cells, then 2 cells into 4, 4 into 8, and so on to create an adult human body with 10 trillion (10×10^{12}) cells. This process is called "ontogeny." Thus, practically all cells in an adult human contain the same 46 chromosomes and similar genetic composition, as all other cells in the body. However, the cells begin to differ in function from one another during embryo development by a process called cell differentiation. The one cell embryo ultimately becomes approximately 200 different types of cells that comprise the tissues and organs of the adult human. This cell differentiation does not involve DNA sequence changes, rather it is achieved by varying the activities (expressions) of the genes (i.e., differential gene regulation/expression) from one cell type to another via a mechanism known as "epigenetics," (described in Chapter 8). Slight changes in the DNA sequence over one's lifetime, due to mutations, has no (or only minor) influences in the cell differentiation process.

(2)   Structure of DNA

The structure of the DNA molecule itself is intriguing. Some of the physical features are described in Chapter 4 and depicted in figure 7.1. Briefly, the DNA in a chromosome actually contains two threads (chains) of a double strand of DNA, each chain comprised of links of sugar molecules with each sugar having an attached molecule called a base. The bases on one thread are paired (connected) to those on the other parallel thread to create a double-stranded DNA in an α-helical conformation. These paired bases are simply referred to as base pairs. In certain locations along the DNA, the sequence of these bases on one thread, contains genetic information to code for proteins, or to code only for RNA (ncRNA). This basic structure is shown in figure 7.1. These protein coding locations (domains) are called "genes" which can transmit genetic information to RNAs with some ultimately coding for proteins. Many additional genes have recently been identified to contain information that codes only for RNA, and not protein (ncRNA). These genes are discussed in more detail below.

Our DNA, and that of all living organisms, has some remarkable physical features. As mentioned earlier in Chapter 4 and listed in table 7.1, and depicted in figure 7.1, each chromosome has one long, helical, double strand of DNA that (when unwound) extends to about 3 to 4 inches. In each of our cells, the 46 chromosomes, combined end to end, would reach 6 feet of double-stranded DNA. As described in Chapter 4 and listed in table 7.1, it is hard to imagine that the total DNA in all 10 trillion (10^{13}) cells in the human body stretches approximately 10 billion miles (or approximately 120 times the distance between the sun and Earth). There are many thousand-fold compactions (approximately a billion fold) of this DNA into the nuclei of cells. This is possible only because the DNA thread in each chromosome is approximately 40 million times longer than it is wide. To add perspective, and as mentioned in Chapter 4, if the width of a DNA strand is enlarged to about ¼ of an inch (about as wide as a pencil), the length of the DNA in each chromosome would stretch to approximately 4,000 miles, a distance longer than the distance between New York and Los Angeles.

For the Human Genome Project, the DNA in all of the chromosomes (the genome), was sequenced to determine the order of the bases along the DNA strand. The sequencing followed these steps: First, the DNA strands (one per chromosome) were unraveled. Second, the bases along the strand were then sequenced in segments and the information for each DNA molecule was stored in computer banks. In total, there are three billion bases (3×10^9) in the 23 single (unpaired) representative chromosomes, which represent the haploid genome.

Figure 7.1

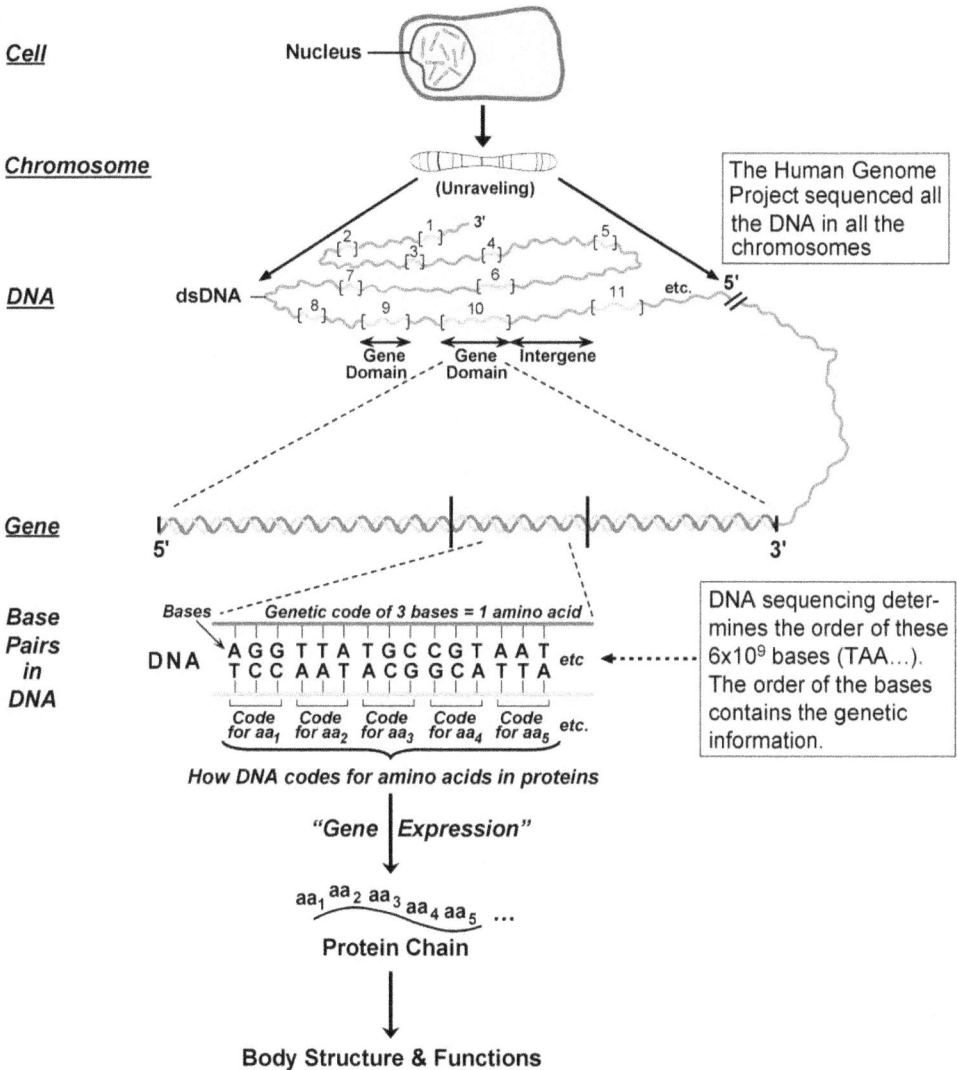

The Human Genome and Genome Project

Cell — Nucleus

Chromosome — (Unraveling)

The Human Genome Project sequenced all the DNA in all the chromosomes

DNA — dsDNA

Gene Domain — Gene Domain — Intergene

Gene — 5' ... 3'

DNA sequencing determines the order of these 6×10^9 bases (TAA...). The order of the bases contains the genetic information.

Base Pairs in DNA

Bases — Genetic code of 3 bases = 1 amino acid

DNA
```
A G G  T T A  T G C  C G T  A A T   etc
T C C  A A T  A C G  G C A  T T A
```
Code for aa_1 Code for aa_2 Code for aa_3 Code for aa_4 Code for aa_5 etc.

How DNA codes for amino acids in proteins

"Gene Expression"

$aa_1 \, aa_2 \, aa_3 \, aa_4 \, aa_5$ ...

Protein Chain

Body Structure & Functions

Figure 7.1 Model of human genome structure illustrating cell, nucleus, chromosomes, and double stranded DNA (dsDNA) with base pairings. The numbers along the DNA strands represent genes numbered in numerical order. The numbers at the end of the DNA strands are a scientific identity of the polarity of the DNA. The aa represents "amino acids."

(Thomas C. Spelsberg and Kenneth Peters, 2011)

Table 7.1

The Astronomical Human Genome and the
Gene Products it Produces

Entity	Number
Cells of the Body:	10 trillion (10^{13})
DNA (length) per cell:	6 feet
Width of DNA:	2×10^{-9} meters
Ratio of DNA Length to Width:	40 million to 1 per chromosome
Total Length of all DNA in Body:	12 billion miles
Genes in a Cell:	20,000 – 25,000
Proteins in a Cell:	60 billion
Species of Protein in the Body:	~100,000
Molecules/Cell:	~10 – 100 trillion ($10^{13} - 10^{14}$)
Molecules/Body:	10^{28} (1 followed by 28 zeros)
Chemical Rx/Cell/Min:	billions

(Thomas C. Spelsberg Ph.D., 2012)

Third, the sequenced data were analyzed by computer programs. This amazing feat initially required 3 billion dollars and 10 years to complete. The sequencing of the 3 billion bases contained enough information to fill 200 large city phonebooks or 2000 computer diskettes. Improved techniques in DNA sequencing, instrumentation, and computer technology were required to achieve this feat. This first whole genome sequence is rather crude (not so accurate) by today's standards. Since then, further improvements in sequencing methodology and computer programming have made the sequencing of genomes of humans, and that of many other living organisms, more accurate, and accomplished faster and cheaper. Today, more accurate and complete sequencing the single human genome can be achieved with several thousand dollars per genome and can be completed in days. Thousands of humans have had their DNA partially sequenced and hundreds have had their genome fully sequenced. The goal of geneticists and the molecular medicine field is to have a complete and accurate genomic analysis available to every human at the cost of $1,000 per genome.

B.   Overview of the Human Genome: Genes, "Junk" DNA, and Non-coding RNAs (ncRNAs)

Many interesting discoveries have been achieved regarding the genomes of humans and other animal, plant, and microbial species. As outlined in tables 7.2, 7.3, and 7.4, one of the amazing discoveries from the early Human Genome Project was the fact that only 1.7-2.0% of the whole genome represents what was termed "functional genes," i.e., regions coding for RNA and, subsequently, proteins which carry out biological functions. Only half of these protein coding genes have been identified with specific functions, i.e., code for proteins with known functions

Table 7.2

Composition of the Human Genome
(From the Human Genome Project)

100% of Genome = ~ 20,000 to 30,000 active genes

⇩

% of the Genome (DNA):

~1.7 - 2.0% = Code for Proteins (~100,000 different types)
(~ Half are of unknown specific function)

~1% = Code for Structural RNAs

~97% = What used to be called Junk DNA (see table 6.3) and is now known to contain:

- Introns (within genes)
- Intergenic regions (between genes)
- Ancient transposable/viral genes (Transporons)
- Ancient/Discarded Genes (Pseudogenes)
- Small regulating RNAs
  In a new breakthrough, it appears that ~70% of junk DNA is transcribed (active); The generated "Small-RNAs" regulate approximately half of the protein coding genes via several mechanisms.

(Thomas C. Spelsberg Ph.D., 2011)

Table 7.3

Detailed Composition of the Human Genome and its Junk DNA as of 2010

DNA Component	% of Total DNA	Characteristics
The Standard DNA Functions		
1. Protein coding genes	2–4%	21,598 genes coding for proteins (enzymes, cell structures, etc.)
2. Non-protein coding regions of genes	20%	Introns, pseudogenes, regulatory domains (enhancers), some microRNAs
3. RNA coding genes tRNA, rRNA	~1%	858 genes involved in protein synthesis and ribosome structure
Composition of the "Junk DNA" as Characterized by Base Sequence (most are functional, i.e., transcriptionally active.)		
4. Small, microRNA coding genes	7-10%	800 microRNA species (genes) (for regulating gene expression)
5. Repeat sequences (indels)	55%	Transposons/retrotransposons, (jumping genes/mobile elements)
a. Long interspersed elements (lines)	40%	850,000 copies (regulates gene expression) (~6.1 kilobase long)
b. Short interspersed elements (sines)	13%	1.5 million copies (regulates gene transcription); Alu sequences
c. Long terminal repeats	1%	
d. DNA transposons	1%	
6. Human endogenous retroviruses	8%	Defective/incomplete viral genome inserts

Data taken from:
Lupski and Stankiewicz (2006); Dudek, R.W. (2010)

Table 7.4

Newest Analyses of the Transcriptionally Active DNA (Active Genes) in the Junk DNA by the ENCODE Project

DNA Component	% of Total DNA	Characteristics
Protein coding genes	~1.7–2.7%	21,000 genes
RNA coding genes	~1.0%	~800 genes - tRNA, ribosomal RNA
Non-protein coding, transcriptionally active regions of the genome	95%	30,000 to 100,000 newly discovered genes actively transcribed
• 8,000 genes coding for small, non- protein coding RNA molecules (SNCs)		Regulating gene expression via mRNA synthesis and turnover and translation
• 9,600 genes coding for long, non-protein coding RNA molecules (LNCs)		Regulating gene expression via mRNA synthesis and turnover and translation
• 11,000 pseudogenes		Some transcriptionally active
• 4 million (4×10^6) small DNA binding elements		Binding regulatory transcription factor proteins (gene regulations)

(Thomas C. Spelsberg Ph.D., 2013)

such as skin protein, muscle protein, connective tissue proteins, and enzymes. Only portions of each protein coding gene domain codes for a protein, and are called the exons. These exon domains of the gene (DNA) are separated by introns, which are domains of a gene which code for RNA but not for the protein. To create a mature, functional messenger RNA (mRNA), the whole gene (all domains) is transcribed into a precursor messenger RNA (pre-mRNA). The intron domains, coded in the pre-mRNA, are removed (spliced) and discarded. The remaining (exon) domains are rejoined as a mature mRNA and translated into protein. This process is called RNA processing. In summary, the protein coding genes in the chromosomes are transcribed in the cell nucleus into pre-mRNA. The pre-mRNA is processed and transported to the cytoplasm and bound to ribosomes. Here the information in the mature mRNA is translated (transferred) into proteins which carry out various functions for the cell.

As mentioned above, the percentage of the protein coding genome represents a surprisingly low value of 20,000–25,000 genes (1.7% of the genome) coding for all the structures that create the complexity of the human body. Scientists are currently focusing on all the exons (i.e., the exome) in all the genes which code for proteins for correlations between polymorphisms and disease. Another 1.0% of the genome is known to code for structural RNAs (called transfer and ribosomal RNAs) which play a role in protein synthesis and cell structures, while the rest of the genome (approximately 97%) was originally termed "junk" DNA. It is now known that, many more domains (now also termed "genes") that code for RNA, but not protein, called non-coding RNA (ncRNA), reside in the junk DNA. These genes are now known to play a role in cell differentiation by regulating gene expression of protein coding genes (epigenetics). Scientists are now elucidating the functions of this "junk" DNA. Table 7.3 and 7.4 outline what is known about this junk DNA composition/function in more detail. We now know that many of these gene sequences in the junk DNA code for non-coding RNA (ncRNA) molecules, which, in turn, regulate the expression of the protein coding genes via a process of "Epigenetic Regulation." This regulation primarily involves the determination of the levels and half-lives of the mRNAs via directing the activities of nuclear exosomes (packets of RNA degrading enzymes) as well as modifying the DNA and histones. These discoveries, generated by recent whole genome sequencing, show the junk DNA region has the following composition:

• Approximately 20% of the junk DNA (approximately 26,000 genes) is ancient, representing inactive genes and active ancient genes, which are classified as pseudogenes.

• A whopping 55% represents repeat sequences caused by ancient viral genomes called transposons and retro-transposons (jumping genes). These cause much of the repeat sequences by duplicating themselves. These ancient viruses infected our human ancestors long ago, some creating multiple interspersed repeat elements. Some of these are transcriptionally active, i.e., produce RNA, as well as play a role in regulating protein gene transcription. When these RNA coding genes are mutated, they cause abnormal protein gene expression and protein production, resulting in diseases.

• Up to 20% or more of the junk DNA represents recently discovered transcriptionally "active" genes, coding for "small" (micro) RNA molecules and long non-protein coding genes (LNCs). These micro- and LNC-nuclear RNAs are classified together as non-coding RNAs (ncRNAs). These genes do not code for (i.e., produce) proteins, but do code for RNA.

These ncRNAs regulate the gene expression of the protein coding genes, mostly via regulating the messenger RNA levels and half-lives, i.e., RNA processing, and ultimately, protein production. They also have recently been shown to play an important role in human diseases.

C.   A New Revelation of Our Genome: "The ENCODE Project Supports That There is No Junk DNA."

In 2012, a $288 million consortium, called the Encyclopedia of DNA Elements (ENCODE) project, funded by the NIH, was created. It is a large group (32 institution and 440 scientist strong), who have combined as the ENCODE group to reassess all the DNA elements in the human genomes using 147 cell types. Their recent findings, reported in 2012 in *Nature and Science*, and outlined in tables 7.3 and 7.4, have shown that 80% to 90% or more of the genome is biologically active, i.e., actively transcribed into RNA. As described above, this project has identified over 30,000 new RNA coding genes (20% of the genome) which code for (transcribe) RNA but do not code for proteins (ncRNAs). Instead, they are involved in both the regulation of the expression of the 20,000 protein coding genes, which represent only 1.7–2.7% of the genome, and possibly also involved in the regulation of each other.

New more definitive studies outlined in table 7.4, resulting from the Encode project, have revealed that "junk" DNA, also contains the following in terms of gene composition:

•   an estimated 8,000 genes represented by small non-protein coding genes coding for microRNA molecules only;

•   an estimated 9,600 genes coding for long (200 base pair) non-protein coding genes (LNC genes) which code only for RNA molecules;

- over 11,000 pseudogenes that were active in the ancient past, some of which are still active or reactivated (transcribing RNA and possibly protein) in some cell types; and finally,

- over 4 million small DNA binding sequences (called regulatory or response elements) which bind regulatory protein transcription factors. These elements (representing approximately 9% of the total genome) are gene switches/ modulators which are bound by the hundreds of regulatory transcription factor (proteins). These elements regulate protein (and possibly non-protein) coding genes.

The active ncRNA coding genes play a major role in the regulating epigenetic processes (i.e., regulating gene activity/transcription) via regulating the mRNA levels and activities. These are further discussed in the next section and in Chapter 8. The transposons (jumping genes) and retrotransposons (causing repeat sequences) represent over half of our genome. As mentioned above, many appear to be the remnants of ancient viral infections (some estimated to be 93 million years old), which have lost their capacity to produce infectious new viruses. Selective sequencing of the active (transcribing) regions of the genome has identified over 100,000 of these viral-like (repeat) DNA sequences (transposons) in the junk DNA of the human genome. Many of these ancient viral genomes have been adopted and used by our cells with some of the genes functioning as "actively expressed" genes. Others duplicate themselves with the replicate inserting into the DNA elsewhere to regulate the protein coding genes. As listed in table 7.5, it is not surprising that mutations in the activities of these repetitive sequences have been found to correlate with certain human diseases.

Table 7.5

Examples of Repeat Sequences associated with Human Disease

<u>ALU Repeats</u>
    Hemophilia
    SCIDs (Immunodeficiency)
    Leukemia
    Autoimmune disease
    Breast cancer
    Neurofibromatosis

<u>Line Repeats</u>
    Hemophilia
    Muscular dystrophy
    β thalassemia
    Retinitis pigmentosa
    Colon cancer
    Chronic granulomatosus

Lupski and Stankiewicz, 2006

Scientists have now identified 200 common diseases caused by mutations, polymorphisms, or abnormal expressions of these repetitive "regulatory" genes in the human junk DNA. All of this new information is truly amazing. It supports that there is no "junk" DNA. However, many areas/elements of the genome are still undefined. The remaining inactive DNA, representing 10% of the genome, may be involved in structural activities (e.g., organization) of the chromosomes.

In any case, one of the early assumptions in biology that "all components of a living cell have a function" is now upheld. It reinforces the theory that life is efficient and doesn't tolerate excess baggage. Importantly, it answers the dilemma that the DNA mutations which have been shown to correlate with human diseases, were found to occur at locations distant from the protein coding genes. Now these DNA changes (also called polymorphisms) make sense as they lie in regulatory genes (i.e., gene switches) which modulate the activities of protein coding genes that are directly involved in diseases.

D.   Comparative Genomics of the Protein Coding Genes: All Life is Genetically Related

Another interesting early discovery from the human genome project was the similarities of the protein coded gene sequences, including their coded protein structure and function, among all living organisms. It has been known for many years that the triplet base alphabet (i.e., the "genetic code" of the DNA) is very similar, among all living things on Earth. Each triplet of bases codes for a specific amino acid (See figure 7.1). Now we know that, among all species of life on Earth, many protein coding genes have similar base sequences as well as their coded protein amino acid sequences. The logic behind these similarities is that the resulting proteins coded by these genes have similar biological functions (both

140

enzymatic and structural) among living organisms. Figure 7.2 shows, as one example, a segment of the human and whale myoglobin. The similarity between the two animal species is remarkable. When one extends these analyses to related genes of other organisms, even more amazing similarities are found.

Figure 7.3 summarizes the protein coding gene sequence similarities of humans to other living organisms such as monkeys, mice, plants, insects, and microbes (yeast, bacteria). Listed in this figure, are the percent of protein coded gene similarities (i.e., base sequence homologies) between human and other living creatures. All humans on Earth display only a 0.1% difference (one base out of a thousand bases difference) in protein coding gene sequences. This represents 3 million variants (differences in base sequence) out of the 3 billion bases of the human haploid genome. As discussed in Chapter 8, these genes are inherited from our parents and their different sequences were caused by natural genetic drift over many thousands of generations. These changes originally occur by random errors in DNA replication over many generations followed by environmental selection for, or against, these errors (Spelsberg, T.C., 2012). In any event, the 95–98% similarity between humans and other primates is not that hard to accept. These few percent difference between humans and monkeys do not seem to be significant. However, they do involve approximately 60 to 150 million base sequence differences per haploid genome between humans and monkeys, involving 80% of the 20–25,000 genes.

Continuing on, it may be hard for one to accept that over 90% of the protein coding genes in rats, mice, dogs, cows, and other mammals are very similar to humans. As an aside, the author's wife refuses to accept that she has 90% genetic similarity to rodents.

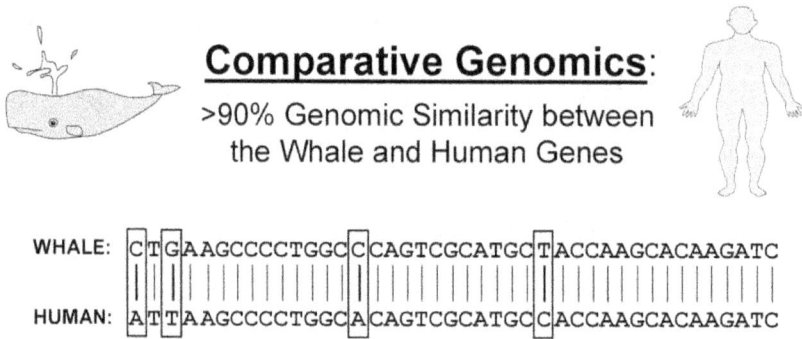

Figure 7.2

Comparative Genomics:
>90% Genomic Similarity between
the Whale and Human Genes

WHALE: CTGAAGCCCCTGGCCCAGTCGCATGCTACCAAGCACAAGATC

HUMAN: ATTAAGCCCCTGGCACAGTCGCATGCCACCAAGCACAAGATC

Figure 7.2 Comparison of the whale and human myoglobin gene domains.

(Thomas C. Spelsberg Ph.D., 2011)

Figure 7.3

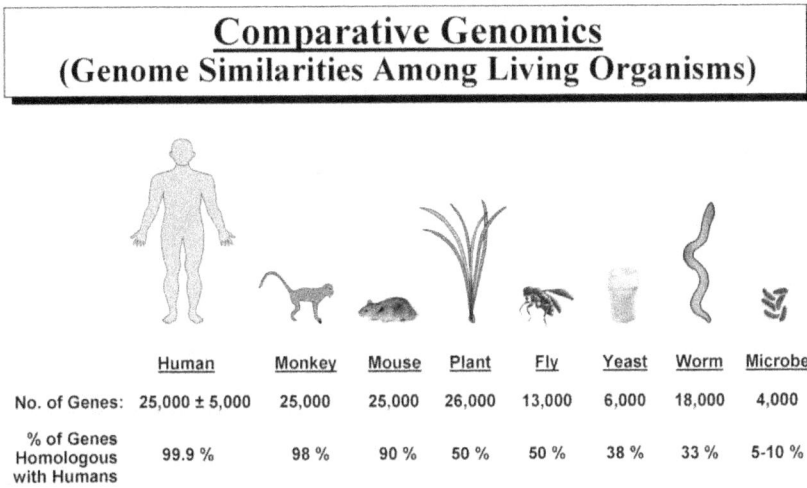

Comparative Genomics
(Genome Similarities Among Living Organisms)

	Human	Monkey	Mouse	Plant	Fly	Yeast	Worm	Microbe
No. of Genes:	25,000 ± 5,000	25,000	25,000	26,000	13,000	6,000	18,000	4,000
% of Genes Homologous with Humans	99.9 %	98 %	90 %	50 %	50 %	38 %	33 %	5-10 %

Figure 7.3 Comparative genomics of living organisms, including gene number and gene homologies compared to the human genome.

(Thomas C. Spelsberg Ph.D., 2011)

Even plants, worms, yeast, and bacterial genes share significant gene similarities with humans. It is interesting to note that our modern human DNA contains Neanderthal and other archaic genes at the level of 2-4%. These are found in European and Asian populations but not Africans. These genes are involved in skin and hair proteins, the immune system, lipid (fat) metabolism, and brain formation. This mating of the archaic humans with modern humans occurred 30-80,000 years ago in the Middle East.

I have often been asked, "What is the rationale for this significant gene similarity among all living things?" As stated above, it is simply that the functions of most of our genes are to carry out basic life processes such as cell replication, cell synthesis of needed cell components, cell repair, energy production, respiration, and metabolism. These are common functions of cells in all living creatures and required for life in general. Thus, the strong genetic similarities among living organisms are due to the fact that many genes are involved in the same basic biological/chemical functions. Differences in many non-protein, RNA coding (ncRNAs) regions (genes) are also somewhat similar (but less identical) across animal species. As discussed earlier, these non-coding genes (coding for ncRNA but not proteins) play a big role in cell differentiation via regulating the activity of protein coding genes by regulating their messenger RNA activities and half-lives by a process called RNA processing, the foundation of "Epigenetics." The pseudogenes, estimated to be 26,000 in humans, are believed to perform similar gene regulatory functions (see table 7.3). The repeat sequences, representing the active transposable elements also play a big role in the epigenetic regulation (of the protein coding genes). As discussed later in Chapter 8, these processes define who each of us are as individuals.

What is so pleasing to the author about these genomic similarities is the realization that there is a strong genetic link among all life on Earth, not only in the genetic code, but gene sequences and protein structures and functions. In short, all life is related. It will be most interesting to learn more about the DNA sequence homologies among all living organisms in all the newly discovered active gene sequences in the junk DNA. On a practical note, it should be mentioned that the significant similarities in gene sequences between humans and other mammals has had major benefits as it has fostered the use of lab animals as models to assess the roles of genes in causing diseases. Scientists can create many human-like diseases in lab animals by disturbing the same genes that are affected in human diseases.

E.   The Story of Telomeres, Aging, Cancer, and Overall Health

(1)   Overview

The story of telomeres is worth mentioning due to their importance. Telomeres are the small sequences at the end of chromosomes that are repeated thousands of times. They are required to prevent the loss of important genes during DNA replication. They are not bound by histones but a special group of non-histone proteins. All living eukaryote cells (e.g., animals, plants, and insects) have telomeres. Telomeres are shortened with every cell division; thus, telomeres lengths shorten as animals/humans (and their cells) age. This is caused by the telomeres enzyme which cannot replicate the far ends of chromosomes. When the telomeres become very short (approximately 1/10–1/100 the original), the cells/animals become "aged" and the cells cease to divide and eventually die. Thus, the number of divisions of all living eukaryote cells is limited, except in the case of cancer cells. It is Mother Nature's natural process of "planned senescence." As discussed below, stem cells and some cancer cells maintain immortalization by sustaining long telomeres.

(2)   Immortalization

Immortalized cells, including embryonic or adult stem cells and cancer cells, have the ability to maintain their telomeres and even lengthen their telomeric DNA. In contrast to normal differentiated cells, most immortalized cells continue to have an active telomerase enzyme that repairs and lengthens the telomeres. In normal, differentiated cells, this activity decreases as the cells age and the telomeres begin to shorten with each cell division. Eventually the cells die. In contrast, immortalized cells maintain long telomeres even after many cell divisions, mostly because they maintain their telomerase activity. This activity is maintained in embryonic and adult stem cells and cancer cells. In fact, scientists have immortalized normal aging adult cells in culture by re-expressing, i.e., reactivating, the telomerase enzyme activity to maintain long telomeres.

(3)   Cancer Exceptions to Telomerase Activation

While most cancer cells are immortalized by activating or maintaining active telomerase enzyme genes, some cancer cells by-pass telomere shortening by unknown mechanisms. Examples of these exceptions are aplastic anemia, acute myeloid leukemia, cancers following Barrett's esophagitis- or ulceritive colitis, epidermal cancers, tongue cancers, and dyskeratosis congenita.

(4)   Shorter Telomeres correlate with Reduced Health and Lifespan

Some recent studies have indicated that older people who have longer telomeres seem to live the longest. People with shorter telomeres die earlier. The latter correlation may be due to a weakened immune system and subsequent infections.

(5)   Childhood Stress causes Shorter Telomeres and Reduced Health and Lifespan

Interesting new studies have provided evidence that stress in childhood, e.g., divorces, single parenthood, poverty, abuse, violence, etc., leads to shortened telomeres. The latter have been shown to correlate with reduced health and lifespan. Mitchell, Notterman, and co-workers, 2014 (P.N.A.S., April 7), reported that stress in boys, especially under 9 years of age, causes a telomere shortening by as much as 40%. Previous studies have demonstrated lesser reductions in telomeres in adults. Now we know that a poor home environment for young children, e.g., violence, lack of direction, family stability, etc., can affect a child's future health, well being, and life expectancy, in addition to the negative effects on their mental disposition.

(6)   Conclusions

The telomeres of our chromosomes shorten in all cells as the cells (and we) age. The exceptions are cancer cells and stem cells which are described in Chapter 11. Thus, telomeres are markers of a cells genetic age and limit the number of replications of each cell. This process prevents old, genetically damaged cells from living on and hurting the whole multicellular organism. The exceptions to these limitations in cell divisions in our bodies are the immortal embryonic and adult stem cells. As we age, the number of stem cells, and thus our ability to repair/regenerate tissues, appear to decrease. Telomeres play a major role in regenerative medicine (Chapters 11 and 12) as they affect not only normal cell aging, including cell death, but also keep stem cells immortal. The accelerated shortening of telomeres by mutations both in the telomere DNA, and in the proteins bound to telomere DNA, have been shown to cause accelerated telomere shortening, early cell death, and premature aging in humans. These alterations have been shown to occur in animals and humans and may play a role in shortened lifespan in such diseases as progeria, as well as in other diseases, e.g., aplastic anemia, pulmonary fibrosis, Alzheimer's, and hepatic cirrhosis.

Alternatively, the sex hormones, especially estrogen, up-regulate telomerase enzyme activity and help maintain telomere length and appear to reduce aging of cells/tissues.

F.   The World of "Omics" - A Brief Description

Since the achievement of the Human Genome Project, many new fields (subfields) have arisen in the world of molecular medicine and biology, and most of these have adopted the "omics" suffix. The author felt it worthwhile to briefly describe some of the more medically relevant terms for the edification of the reader. Some of these are listed in table 7.6. The suffix "omics" is used for fields of study such as genomics, proteomics, etc. The prefix is used to identify the objects being studied or referred to; examples are gen(ome), prote(ome), and microbi(ome). There are currently over 400 accepted technical terms using the "omics" suffix.

G.   Why So Few Genes for Such a Complex Organism?

What is also amazing is the fact that the human body is extremely complex. As discussed in Chapter 4, there are, in each of us, ten trillion cells (10×10^{12} cells) that are specialized into approximately 200 different cell types. There are actually a much greater number of subtypes of cells with specific functions. Each cell has millions of chemical reactions occurring every minute. It is also fascinating that all these cells and their molecules act in a coordinated pattern with each other to

Table 7.6

Examples of Medical/Biological Fields involving "Omics"

I. Genomics: Study of the genomes of organisms.
    a. Cognitive genomics: Examines the changes in cognitive processes associated with genetic profiles.
    b. Comparative genomics: Studies of the relationship of genome structure and function across different biological species or strains
    c. Functional genomics: Examines gene and protein functions and interactions
    d. Metagenomics: Studies the metagenomes (i.e., genetic material) that are present in environmental samples.
    e. Personal genomics: Branch of genomics concerned with the sequencing and analysis of the genome of an individual.
    f. Epigenomics: The study of the complete set of epigenetic modifications on the genetic material of a cell, known as the epigenome.
    g. Transcriptomics: The study of the transcriptome is the set of all RNA molecules, including mRNA, rRNA, tRNA, and other non-coding RNA produced in one or a population of cells.

II. Proteomics: The study of the proteome, i.e., the entire complement of proteins, particularly their structures and functions, including the modifications made to a particular set of proteins in an organism or system.
III. Metabolomics is the scientific study of chemical processes involving metabolites. It is a "systematic study of the unique chemical fingerprints that specific cellular processes leave behind", the study of their small-molecule metabolite profiles.
IV. Nitrogenomics: Study of the effects of foods and food constituents on gene expression. Studies the effect of nutrients on the genome, proteome, and metabolome.
V. Pharmacogenomics investigates the effect of the sum of variations within the human genome on drugs.
VI. Pharmacomicrobiomics investigates the effect of variations of the human microbiome on drugs.
VII. Toxicogenomics: A field of science that deals with the collection, interpretation, and storage of information about gene and protein activity within particular cell or tissue of an organism in response to toxic substances.
VIII. Psychogenomics: Process of applying the powerful tools of genomics and proteomics to achieve a better understanding of the biological substrates of normal behavior and of diseases of the brain that manifest themselves as behavioral abnormalities.
IX. Stem cell genomics: Helps in stem cell biology. Aim is to establish stem cells as a leading model system for understanding human biology and disease states.

Taken from Wikipedia.org - The free encyclopedia ("Omics" – Wikipedia.Wikimedia Foundation, April 1, 2013) maintain life. How could all this complexity arise from only 20,000–25,000 genes? This discrepancy can be explained by three processes: First, each gene often codes for multiple products (RNA and proteins); second, these thousands of protein products function in various combinations with each other; and third, the expression (activity) of each gene is regulated differently among different cell types and living species by "Epigenetic" processes. The protein coding genes often produce several to many different proteins by changing the start and stop sites for messenger RNA synthesis; differential splicing of introns, and differential translation (protein synthesis) start and stop sites on the messenger RNAs by the ribosomes. Together, the inheritance of altered genes from our parents combined with the above processes, give rise to individualism in each of us (e.g., differences in appearance, in physical and metabolic characteristics, and disease predisposition).

The role of epigenetics involves both long-term and short-term regulation of gene expression without altering the DNA (gene) sequence. As outlined in the next chapter, this regulation involves:

• actions of the thousands of non-coding RNAs (ncRNAs);

• chemical modifications, e.g., phosphorylations and acetylations, of the inhibitory histones which cover the DNA (genes) in chromosomes;

• the actions of the transcription factor proteins which bind to their DNA elements near genes along with their chemical modifications; as well as

• the chemical modifications of the DNA (e.g., DNA methylation) that inhibits or activates gene activity.

These functions markedly increase the complexities of gene expression, leading to millions of possibilities, and thus, account for the complexity of the human body and the creation of each of human (and animal) as an individual. The inherited unique DNA sequences and epigenetic mechanisms in our genomes represent the primary cause of why we are each individuals: metabolically, physically, including drug metabolism, personalities, and disease predispositions. The epigenetic mechanisms explain why even identical twins become more non-identical as they age.

Chapter 8

How Genes and Epigenetics Create the Human Individual

Definitions

chromosome: structures in the cell nucleus that contain DNA (genes) and associated proteins. There are 46 chromosomes in most cells of the human body.

DNA methylation: methylation of cytosine in/around gene domains that can restrict gene activity (gene expression); involved in the epigenetic regulation of gene expression.

environment-induced mutations: DNA (gene) mutations and possibly epigenetic changes caused by environmental mutagens such as chemicals and ultraviolet light, and atomic radiation. Examples of such environmental mutagens are cigarette smoking, coal dust, and sunlight.

epigenetics: (meaning "above Genetics"); the study of factors and processes that influence (regulates) gene expression, but do not alter the genotype (DNA sequence); the regulation of gene expression (RNA and protein production) by mechanisms other than changes in the DNA; examples are: DNA modifications (methylation), histone and transcription factor modifications (acetylation, phosphorylation), and microRNA regulation of protein synthesis and mRNA stability; current analyses of epigenetic effects are measurements of mRNA and protein levels and enzyme activities.

genetic drift: periodic, spontaneous changes over time and generations in human (and animal) DNA; ultimately can cause changes in the appearance and physiology over many generations in isolated populations via environmental selection creating ethnic groups in humans, and thus, does play a major role in creating individuals by the inheritance of unique genes from parents; different animal species can evolve if the drift occurs over very long periods; since the mutations, environmental selection, and subsequent appearance of polymorphisms, due to genetic drift, occur at a very slow but relatively constant frequency; these polymorphisms can be applied to genetic tracking of human origins and world migrations.

genetic (parental) imprinting: expression of genes is determined by the parent who contributed them: one of the pair of genes (either one from the mother or one from the father) is expressed; the other is repressed.

histone modification: side chain modification of histone proteins by acetylation, methylation, phosphorylation, and ubiquitination, which affects DNA condensation and gene expression; involved in epigenetic regulation of gene expression.

identical twins (monozygotic twins): twins which arise from the division of the same fertilized egg to create two distinct embryos with identical sets of inherited genes.

long non-coding RNAs (lncRNAs): long non-coding RNAs that regulate the protein synthesis of coding messenger RNA similar to microRNAs; a subclass of ncRNAs.

meiosis: single whole nuclear (DNA) duplication in a precursor diploid germ cell followed by two successive nuclear divisions creating the haploid germ cells (sperm or egg) with half the normal set of 23 unpaired chromosomes.

microRNAs: subclass of ncRNAs; small non-coding RNAs each of which have different classes/functions; one primary function is to carry out epigenetic (gene) regulation by binding to mRNAs, preventing protein synthesis and encouraging the mRNA degradation; these small RNAs fine tune the mRNA levels and thus gene expression without altering the DNA (gene) sequence.

mitosis: the total chromosome duplication followed by a single division of a diploid (somatic) cell resulting in two identical cells each of which has the normal (diploid) number of 46 chromosomes; occurs in many adult cells/tissues in the human body throughout a lifetime.

single nucleotide polymorphisms (SNPs): changes of a single base nucleotide in the DNA found in the human genome.

transposable elements (transposons/jumping genes): class of DNA sequences that replicates itself with the new DNA copy moving from one chromosome domain to another or from chromosome to chromosome; there are several subclasses of this class, often creating repeat sequences and affecting gene expression by inserting its copy near a gene to regulate its transcription.

A.   Introduction

We realize by just observing fellow humans around us, that we are each unique individuals. This is routinely reinforced by the rarity found in tissue matches for organ transplants. This chapter describes how we become unique individuals. The creation of the individual is globally defined under the process, "Ontogeny." It involves: 1) the unique genes carried by each family which will be inherited; 2) the redistribution of these genes during sperm and egg production; 3) the selection of which sperm and egg used for each fertilization; and 4) the regulation of the expression of these genes in the embryo and subsequent adult by a process of epigenetics that continues throughout one's lifetime. The creation of the individual is Mother Nature's plan to allow living entities to adapt and survive. Unfortunately it also leads to diseases such as cancer. One of the best known processes that create individual traits is the inheritance of unique genes which arise over many generations via genetic drift.

B.   Creating Individualism by the Unique Genes We Inherit

A brief description of "genetic drift," which contributes to both ethnic and individual population traits over long periods (thousands of years), is warranted. These traits are due, in part, to the unique genes we inherit from our parents. Keep in mind, the original genome of living prokaryote organisms originated approximately 3.8 billion years ago, and the eukaryote organism originated approximately 2.0 billion years ago. These genomes have undergone numerous changes during evolution over billions of years, due to a process called genetic drift. Genetic drift begins with the rare DNA mutations that occur periodically and spontaneously in the human genome as errors in DNA replication. These are mostly represented as changes in single nucleotide (base) sequences, but can involve additions, deletions, or rearrangements of larger segments of the DNA. These errors are originally caused by the DNA replication enzyme (DNA polymerase) that operates very rapidly (up to 1000 bases polymerized per second) and occasionally makes random errors that ultimately create "mutations" (approximately 1 out of 10,000—100,000 bases in the DNA). The cell has DNA repair mechanisms which repair most, but not all, of these errors, resulting in only approximately 100 base mutations remaining after each genome replication of 6 billion bases in the diploid (somatic) cell. These 100 errors from each cell division represent 1/100,000 percent (0.00001%) or 1 out of 30 million base pairs of the haploid genome. These accumulating spontaneous, random errors are passed on to the offspring via sperm and egg as mutations. The frequencies of these changes (mutations) in the human genome are amplified by environmental selection of the population and accumulate over many generations. As a result of environmental selection, some mutations occasionally expand to 1% of a population, which then, for convenience sake, scientists reclassify as polymorphisms. See the book by T. C. Spelsberg, "The Myth of Race," 2011, for simple explanations.

To summarize, the DNA polymorphisms (changes in base sequences), which accumulated over thousands to millions of years, create unique individual genomes (i.e., genes) with an enormous number of unique polymorphism patterns in the genes in the human population. Today, an average of about 1 out of every 1000 bases, representing 6 million (or 0.1%) of the total 6 billion DNA bases of a diploid cell, differ between one human and another. Remember, this value represents the accumulated changes over many generations. The rare DNA mutations that occur during a single lifetime only play a minor role in creating each of us as individuals. However, these errors accumulate and their effects multiply over many lifetimes. The individual differences in DNA base sequences (genes) have now increased to about 1 base difference out of 1000 from one individual to another. This represents 3 million base pair differences per haploid cell genome or 6 million base pair differences per diploid cell genome. These are the unique genes we inherit from our parents.

It is important to mention that similar errors also occur during the replication of DNA in the mitochondria of human cells. The frequency of such changes (errors) in mitochondria is 10 times the frequency of errors in chromosomal DNA and is known to cause approximately 2 dozen human diseases. These mitochondrial DNA errors also accumulate over generations to create individual patterns. When an excess of DNA mutations occurs in the mitochondria, they are discarded by the cells phagosomes. Remember, the mitochondrial diseases are inherited from the mothers because only females can pass mitochondria to offspring. Similarly, diseases due to errors in the Y chromosome are inherited only from the father.

C.   Creating Individualism by the Random Redistribution of Maternal and Paternal Genes during Sperm and Egg Production

(1)   Overview

As outlined in table 8.1 and described above, genetic drift, over long periods, not only causes physical/metabolic changes in populations/ethnic groups, but plays a role in the creation of unique genes. Thus, we inherit our individual traits by the inheritance of these unique gene sequences. These unique genes are the cause of many of the physical and metabolic differences, including diseases, observed between individuals and ethnic groups. As described next, these unique genes are then markedly redistributed during meioses by chromosome exchange

Table 8.1

**Physiological Differences among Individuals from
Europe, Africa, China, and Japan**

A. Continent-specific physiology/developmental functions:

Skeletal/muscular system   Digestive system
Connective tissue   Cardiovascular system
Hair and skin   Drug metabolism

B. Continent-specific diseases/disorders

Metabolism   Cancer   Immunological
Reproduction   Blood

- -

However, over time, individuals within each population display up
to six times greater differences among each other than those that
exist among populations. This is due to continuing spontaneous
genetic changes in each individual.

"Thus, the new field of "Individualized Medicine"

(Data taken from Baye et al, 2009, and Bar-bujani et al, 1997) during egg and sperm production, after which the chromosomes are randomly dispersed to each sperm and egg. These processes are the cause of the inheritance of unique sets of genes in each offspring. This creates individual differences among all animals, including humans, and plants and insects. Tables 8.2 and 8.3, and the next section, outline the gene rearrangements that occur in each human genome during sperm/egg production and the final selection of which sperm fertilizes which egg. These processes, causing human/animal individuality and diversification and individualism, in addition to our inherited unique genes, are Mother Nature's way of generating diversity and environmental adaptation for survival's sake. Sadly, these survival strategies occasionally cause diseases such as cancer in some individuals.

(2)   Individualism due to Chromosome Recombination and Redistribution of Unique Parental Genes during Formation of Germ Cells (Sperm and Egg)

Germ cells (sperm and egg), each containing half of a person's genome, join together to create the fertilized egg, which contains a complete genome. The germ cells are, in turn, created through meiosis. Meiosis is a complex process involving the following events:

• chromosome/DNA replication in a pre-germ cell;

• exchange of common large segments between the father's and mother's paired chromosomes; (i.e., termed "genetic recombination" or "crossing over" of the DNA strands between chromosomes); this exchange, termed "crossing over," of large DNA segments between the paired chromosomes, each with their unique sets of the father's and mother's genes, occurs in both the sperm and egg

Table 8.2

List of the Various Processes involved in Altering the Genetic Make-up to Create an Individual

A. The Genome

- Age: approximately 3.8 billion years

- Composition (DNA): Same among all life forms

- Genetic code (information): Basically identical among all life forms

B. Individual genomic changes during an individual's lifetime (from the sperm/unfertilized egg to end of life)

- Copy errors during replication
  Fixed single base changes
  Insertions and deletions (indels)
  Tandem duplication

- Homologous recombination (chromosomal)
  Exchanges in similar long segments (chromosome crossovers)

- Random distribution of the chromosomes into the sperm/egg

- Genetic (parental) imprinting
  Selecting whether the father's or mother's paired gene will be expressed (epigenetics)
- Transposable elements
  Ancient viral life sequences that replicate and insert their sequences at various places around the genome (adding DNA to genome)

- New viral infections
  Many viruses infect living host cells (including bacteria) and insert their genomes into the host's genome

- Rearrangements creating:
  Inversions, deletions, duplications (copy no. variants)

- Whole chromosome fusions, fissions, and translocations (e.g., attached Y chromosomes, and trisomy 21)

- Whole genome duplication within the same cell

- Epigenetic (somatic) changes in gene expression via differential gene regulation (e.g., histone/DNA modifications, transcription factors, and microRNA actions on messenger RNAs)

- Transposon activities regulating gene expression

- Environmental (physical or chemical) induced genetic changes [e.g., smoking, air pollution, radiation (sun), chemical exposure]

(Thomas C. Spelsberg Ph.D., 2013)

Table 8.3

Biological Processes in Addition to Genetic Inheritance which are involved in Creating an Individual Human (as per the Stage of Human Development)

A. Sperm/Egg Formation

   1. Recombination: The crossing over (exchange) of chromosomal segments, exchanging DNA each with unique DNA changes, i.e., polymorphisms

   2. Random distribution of newly constructed chromosomes into sperm or eggs

B. Fertilization and Embryo

   1. Parental (genetic) imprinting

   2. Chromosome rearrangement (translocations, fusions, deletions, inversions)

   3. Epigenetic activities

      a. Histone modifications

      b. Chemical modifications of the DNA

      c. Modifications of transcription factors

      d. Modifications by microRNAs and long non-coding RNAs

      e. Jumping genes (transposons)

C. Post-natal Development and Aging

   1. Continuation of epigenetic changes

   2. Environmental induced genetic changes

(Thomas C. Spelsberg Ph.D., 2013)

production. This process is also termed "recombination." This strand exchange generates an enormous variety in the offspring with a minimal estimate of over 8 million possible exchange locations among all the paired chromosomes. Combining both the sperm and egg, there are 70 trillion possible variations in the embryo;

• two cell divisions which include the random separation of each of the paired chromosomes create intact, complete half sets of chromosomes (haploid) for each sperm cell (sperm and egg); and finally,

• the distribution of the final processed chromosomes of each pair into each sperm or egg is random, further mixing the father's and mother's chromosomes.

Through these mechanisms, no two germ cells (sperm/egg) and offspring are exactly the same among the billions of sperm or eggs, with each representing unique mixtures of unique genes in both maternal and paternal lineages. The exception to the above is identical twins that come from the same fertilized egg (thus avoiding the variations of the chromosome exchanges and selections). Identical twins start life as an embryo with the same genetic makeup. This includes the maternal and paternal chromosomal exchanges and distribution. However, it should be mentioned that even twins will not remain identical during the subsequent development and aging due to the epigenetic regulation of gene expression. This process begins even *in utero* as embryos develop. The story of identical twins is described later in this chapter.

(3)   Individualism due to the Random Selection of which Sperm and Egg Fertilize

The final determination of the inheritance of an individual involves the selection of which of the millions of sperm will actually fertilize which egg. The resulting fertilized egg is diploid, with one set of genes (alleles) from the mother, and one set of genes (alleles) from the father.

D.   Creating Individualism after Fertilization by Epigenetics (The Regulation of Gene Expression)

   (1)   Introduction

The final significant mechanism involved in creating individual traits is the differential regulation of gene expression (RNA and protein synthesis) in the embyro, the baby, and the adult individual. This process is the basis of a new scientific field called "epigenetics." Major differences between human individuals, including identical twins, are now believed to be caused by this differential expression of genes. Epigenetics is currently measured by determining gene expression patterns, e.g., mRNA, protein, and/or enzyme activity levels. These genetic regulatory mechanisms involve non-DNA (non-genomic) alterations in the chromosomes (see table 8.4 and figure 8.1). These processes are the major forces involved in cell differentiation and organism development (i.e., ontogeny), and create rapid and permanent differences between individual humans. Similar epigenetic mechanisms occur in plants, insects, and animals. Epigenetics is the foundation of genetic (parental) imprinting such as determining which of the two homologous genes (alleles) or whole X chromosome in females (one from the mother and one from the father) will be expressed and the other repressed.

As mentioned above, even identical twins, as they age, display ever increasing differences in appearance, disease predispositions, and metabolism due to epigenetics. However, as mentioned above, identical twins start out and remain more genetically identical than non-identical twins and other siblings.

Table 8.4

Processes that Regulate Gene Expression: Genomic and Non-Genomic (Epigenetic) Mechanisms

A. Regulation via Altering the Genotype (Polymorphisms)

Changes in the DNA sequence which alters the gene expression +

- Single nucleotide changes

- Excision/additions of DNA segments, including transposons, viruses

B. Epigenetics: Regulation of Gene Expression via Non-Genomic Processes

Target	Inhibiting Gene Expression	Enhancing Gene Expression
• DNA	Methylation	De-methylation
• Histone	Methylation	De-methylation
• Histone	De-acetylation	Acetylation
• Histone	De-phosphorylation	Phosphorylation
• Transcription Factor	Suppressor	Activator
• MicroRNA/Long non-coding RNAs	Yes	Yes
• Transposons (jumping genes) and retrotransposons	Yes	Yes

(Thomas C. Spelsberg Ph.D., 2013)

Figure 8.1

Epigenetic Processes in Gene Expression

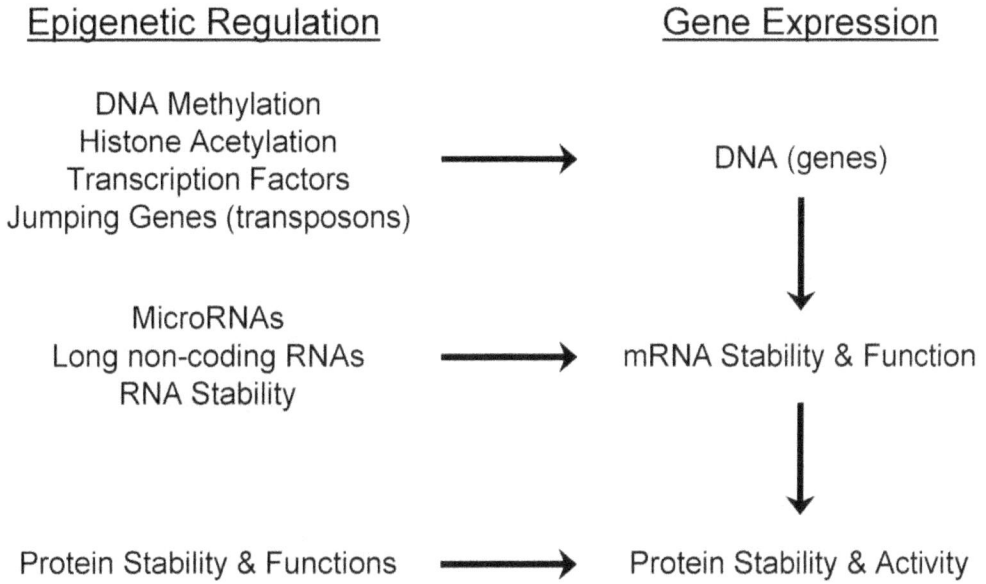

<u>Epigenetic Regulation</u>   <u>Gene Expression</u>

DNA Methylation
Histone Acetylation
Transcription Factors   ⟶   DNA (genes)
Jumping Genes (transposons)
                                                                    ↓

MicroRNAs
Long non-coding RNAs   ⟶   mRNA Stability & Function
RNA Stability
                                                                    ↓

Protein Stability & Functions   ⟶   Protein Stability & Activity

Identical twins arise after the fertilized egg divides and the many possible variables in DNA polymorphisms and gene distribution have already been established. The fertilized egg thus gives rise to two identical twin offspring. However, as discussed discussed below, identical twins begin to differ over time as soon as they are created, as a result of epigenetic processes.

There are multiple mechanisms involved in the differential regulation of gene expression/activity (epigenetics) which contribute to human individualism. These are outlined in tables 8.2, 8.3, 8.4, and figure 8.1. When a single celled fertilized embryo divides into 2 cells, and those 2 cells divide into 4, and so on, hundreds of times, 200 cell types and 10 trillion (10^{13}) cells ultimately create the human body. This developmental process is known as "Ontogeny." This complex process is possible by the differential (epigenetic) expression of the 20,000 or so protein coding genes (and possibly ncRNA genes). Their protein products then interact in different combinations with each other to create a multitude of different functions. Further, the RNA coding genes in the "junk DNA," which code for the non-coding RNA (ncRNA), also display altered (regulated) activities and thus differentially regulate the expression of the protein coding genes via epigenetic processes. These processes ultimately create different cell types (cell differentiation) and the individual with his/hers specific disease predisposition, personality, tissue antigens, and metabolism. These constant changes in individuals, combined with environmental selection, improve the species, so that some can adapt to challenges of a constantly changing environment in order for the species to survive.

Regulating gene expression by the processes of epigenetics, in a way, is safer as it is reversible, since it does not involve permanent changes in the DNA (genetic information) and it occurs at a more rapid rate. Epigenetics is rapidly reversible compared to the processes involved in changing the genetic information in the DNA itself, which is more permanent. Epigenetics has opened the door to a whole new world of medical research. The following sections briefly describe each of the various mechanisms involved in epigenetics, i.e., the regulation of genes. These represent several specific, well documented mechanisms of epigenetic regulation of gene expression that are major contributors of individualism among humans, including all other multicellular eukaryote organisms. These are outlined in table 8.2 and figures 8.1 and 8.3.

(2)   Epigenetic Gene Regulation by Chemically Modifying the DNA: New Studies in the Brain and Behavior

The DNA nucleotides (bases) in the DNA can be enzymatically methylated or demethylated by enzymes to inhibit or activate gene expression respectively. The methylation of the bases usually represses the rate of gene expression/transcription, while the demethylation of the DNA bases will activate/enhance gene expression. Keep in mind, the DNA sequence (i.e. genetic information in base sequences) is not altered in these epigenetic processes; only reversible chemical side changes of the bases occur. The methylation and demethylation of the DNA is readily reversible by enzymes (methylases and demethylases), and thus can rapidly change the state of gene expression. It should be mentioned that other chemical modifications of the bases also occur in epigenetics. Scientists at the John's Hopkins Medical Center have shown that the extent of DNA methylation in blood cells correlates with, and possibly even causes, severe mood changes and post-partum depression. As discussed later in this chapter, others have found that DNA methylation plays a role in the development of synapses between neurons in animal/human brains and thus, a role in behavior.

(3)   Epigenetic Regulation by Chemically Modifying DNA Bound Histones: Roles in Memory and Autism

To create "chromatin," all eukaryotes (plants, animals, insects, and fungi) have positively charged proteins (histones) bound to negatively charged DNA to partially fold the DNA into "nucleosomes" which are spherical structures. These histones can more extensively fold (x 10,000 fold) the chromatin/DNA into compact bodies known as "chromosomes." These histones are highly conserved over evolution and help protect the DNA, maintain order and structure, and assist in the regulation of gene expression. To accomplish the latter, the histones are often enzymatically modified by small organic molecules, e.g., acetyl, methyl, phosphatyl, or ubiquitin groups, which reduce their binding to DNA, causing them to release the DNA, resulting in the activation of gene expression. This chemical modification of histones is rapidly reversible, which again allows a rapid inhibition of gene expression as non-modified histones.

In studies to retrieve memories and enhance learning in lab animals, scientists found that drugs that enhance the histone acetylation activates gene expression in the brain. Dr. Tsai and colleagues at MIT, Dr. Wood and colleagues at the University of California-Irvine, and Dr. Sweatt at the University of Alabama-Birmingham, have used these drugs to enhance not only animal learning and memories, but also to help humans with autism, Alzheimer's, and other age-related senility. It is now known that the number of brain neuron connections is increased when the histone acetylation in the brain is activated by these drugs, which, in turn, enhances gene expression. Enzymes, that deacetylate the histones, repress gene expression and are speculated to reduce memory, learning, and increase senility.

(4)   Epigenetic Regulation by Transcription Factor Proteins and Growth Factor/Cytokines

Another well documented epigenetic mechanism involves the actions of "transcription factors," proteins that regulate the expression of genes by binding to specific elements nearby the genes (see figure 8.1). The classes of these factors, their concentrations, and their level of activity, in turn, are also regulated by chemical modifications, e.g., phosphorylation. These factors determine which genes are regulated, when and how they are regulated, increased or decreased, and to what extent. An extended family of this group codes for growth factors and cytokines, which are protein factors that indirectly regulate gene transcription. These protein factors are secreted from one cell and bind to the membrane receptors of neighboring or distant cells. Once connected to target cells, they activate or inhibit signaling pathways that extend into the nucleus to regulate the genes of these cells. The result of this class of regulatory factors is the better coordination of efforts among the cells and tissues of the whole body. These protein factors are highly conserved over evolution.

(5)   Epigenetic Regulation by MicroRNAs and Long Non-coding RNAs

As briefly described in Chapter 7, a sizable portion of our genome is now known to code for non-coding RNAs (ncRNAs) which do not code for proteins. These ncRNAs include small RNAs (microRNAs) and long non-coding RNAs (lncRNAs). Studies of small nuclear RNAs and their biological functions began over 30 years ago (Lerner et al, 1980; Wieben et al, 1983). In the past decade, some of these microRNAs have been shown to bind to the DNA to regulate transcription (i.e., the rate of RNA synthesis). However, most of these microRNAs are now known to bind to messenger RNAs (mRNA) to inhibit their translation into proteins or to limit their half-life (see figure 8.1) (Lago-Quintana, et all, 2001). Thus, this process regulates gene expression mainly at the level of mRNA stability and protein synthesis. Currently, there are about 8000 known microRNA species presumably transcribed from 8000 distinct genes located in the classical junk DNA domain (see table 7.4). These numbers are assuredly low with estimates of as many as 50,000 such RNA species and their genes in existence. The role of these microRNAs in creating differences among human individuals, including physical development and metabolic functions, etc., is only now being elucidated. These RNAs are involved in regulating (usually repressing) gene expression both at the gene transcription and protein production levels. Currently much is being learned about the regulation of multiple gene expressions by these microRNAs, the various steps/processes involved, and their relationships to diseases.

Recently, the long lncRNAs found in the nucleus have also been shown to regulate the expression of genes. These lncRNAs are coded by genes located near the genes they regulate. Some (possibly all) of these belong to a class of genes called pseudogenes. These RNAs usually repress gene transcription/ expression. It is important to note that the complexity of our gene regulation increases enormously when one considers that the levels/activities of the lncRNAs and the microRNAs are themselves regulated.

(6)   Epigenetic Regulation by Jumping Genes (Transposable Elements): Actions in Brain Development, Senility, Learning, Disposition, and Autism

Recently, a novel role for jumping genes (sometimes called transposons or transposable elements) in epigenetic regulation has been identified. These genes were first discovered by Barbara McClintock over 60 years ago. Initially, she received much opposition and criticism for her work. Transposons are suspected to be involved in changes in the appearance, metabolism, disposition and disease predisposition among individuals, including identical twins. While this process does not alter the specific DNA (gene) sequence, it does alter gene/DNA internal arrangements and often causes a change in expression of nearby genes.

Transposons are long and short interspersed DNA elements, flanked by repeat sequences, which have been inserted into the genome by viruses. Some of these viruses appear to have infected our ancestors as early as 93 million years ago and have been active in our primate ancestors ever since. Some of these were then adapted by our cells to regulate gene expression. Ancient viral genomes now make up over half of the human genome and some behave as newly acquired genes. Most of these genes are located in the "junk DNA." Some of these sequences jump from one location to another (transposons), some carrying along genes located nearby. Others first replicate and reinsert an identical copy elsewhere in our DNA (transposons and retrotransposon). This replication process increases the size of our genome. When these transposons insert their DNA segments near genes, they can cause differential regulation of gene expression. This activity adds to the uniqueness of individuals, including disease susceptibility. Recent studies have revealed that the average individual human brain cell has over 7500 copies of just one type of transposon elements. In addition, there are over 10,000 copies of just one type of retrotransposons at various locations in the human genome.

It is important to distinguish the two types of jumping genes: "Transposons" which usually leave one location and insert themselves into another location on the

DNA/chromosomes and only sometimes will duplicate themselves; and "retrotransposons" which are DNA elements which are transcribed into RNA, but with the original DNA remaining at the original location. This RNA is then transcribed back into DNA to be reinserted elsewhere in the genome. This is how these jumping genes create multiple copies of additional identical sequences (i.e., repeat sequences) and enlarge the genome. The important epigenetic aspect of these jumping genes is that they regulate protein coding genes. These transposons and retrotransposons are active throughout one's lifetime in practically all cells of the body, and they are suspected to play a role in the differentiation of progenitor (stem) cells into many cell types. A few transposons have recently been shown to be transcribed into RNA and proteins of unknown functions.

In recent studies, scientists at the Salk Institute and the University of California recently reported that transposons are especially active in stem (progenitor) cells of many adult tissues, e.g., the neurons in the hippocampus and caudate nucleus of the brain, in the ovaries, and in the testes. It was found that a high level of jumping gene activity occurs early in the developing brain. This activity continues into adulthood of lab animals, and is enhanced when the animals are "learning." Recently, scientists at the Roslin Institute in Scotland and the Salk Institute in California reported that the activities of these jumping genes (transposons) may be involved in creating different personalities/dispositions, including responses to stress, moods, and behavior. Some of these effects of transposons in the brain can last a lifetime. Overall, scientists now think that transposon activity not only causes randomly different behaviors and dispositions, but also is involved in learning processes and memory.

As mentioned earlier, the insertion of these elements not only regulates the activity (up or down) of nearby protein coding genes, but they also can create variants of a protein by inserting themselves inside the gene coding for a specific protein. These events either help a cell/organism or hurt it, e.g., cause diseases such as cancer, autism, etc. In any case, their purpose for Mother Nature is to cause rapid changes that allow the organism to meet the demands of adaptation and survival. The cells and organs (e.g., brains) of one human individual will have different levels of activity and patterns of insertions of transposons compared to another human individual, thus creating individual differences in gene expression, personalities/dispositions, mental and metabolic diseases, and possibly mental abilities. Scientists have recently reported that these jumping genes appear to play a role in autism, Crohn's disease, schizophrenia, and senility. Dr. Kato and colleagues at the Riken Brain Institute in Waco City, Japan, have reported that jumping genes cause or contribute to schizophrenia. Gage and colleagues at the University of California, San Diego, have shown that well known jumping gene, called L1, is abundant in human stem cells in the brain and plays a role in neuron development and mental disorders, e.g., Rett syndrome (autism) and Louis-Bar syndrome.

Jumping gene activity occurs in all cells of the body. This activity begins when we are embryos and continues throughout life. In addition to the chemical modifications of the DNA and histones, the transposons and retrotransposons are now thought to help create differences in physical appearances, metabolism, learning capabilities, memory, personality dispositions, tissue/organ compatibilities, and disease predisposition among individuals, even between siblings and identical twins.

E.   The Story of Identical Twins

As stated earlier, identical twins begin embryonic life with an identical inherited genome (i.e., identical genes with identical patterns of polymorphisms). Even though they began with identical genomes, eliminating the differences in inherited genes from germ cells, changes in gene expression (epigenetics) in identical twins begin right after each embryo is formed. These changes continue through embryonic, perinatal, and adult life. If each twin is truly identical to the other, when one twin has a disease such as schizophrenia, bipolar disorder, major depression, or autism, one would expect that the other would surely develop the disease as well (i.e., 100% chance). However, clinical studies show that the other twin has only a 40–50% chance of getting these diseases. Non-identical twins and other siblings show only a 10–30% correlation in these diseases among each other. Non-related individuals show even less (<1–10%) correlation. Personality traits and preferences, such as homosexuality, are similarly different (40–50%) between identical twins. Identical twins display unique differences even in fingerprints. Recent studies by Craig and colleagues at the Murdoch Children's Research Institute in Australia, have demonstrated that the major cause of twin differences, which cannot be different due to different genes inherited from parents, is due to the rapid epigenetic regulatory pattern differences.

It needs to be reminded that identical twins will generate specific minor changes in their individual genomes during their lifetime as a result of genetic drift, due to spontaneous replication errors, and occasional environment induced changes. This is negligible when compared to the 6 billion bases in our diploid genome. More profound are the effects of the above described epigenetic processes in cells and tissues, including the brains of adult identical twins. The environment and other influences also contribute to individual differences between twins, by altering the epigenetics. Examples of the latter include twin differences in nourishment *in utero*, as well as differences during the life of identical twins in diet and behavior, such as smoking. In support of this view, the correlations of disease occurrences are closer when identical twins grow up together (i.e., in the same environment and with the same habits), compared to instances where they grow up separately or expose themselves to different environments, including diets, etc. To quote Dr. Champagne of Columbia University, "As you walk through life and have unique experiences, your epigenetic changes often reflect these changes."

F.   What is a Predisposition for a Disease?

Disease predisposition is an individual trait and sometimes a family trait. Having a predisposition for a disease means that there is a greater than a random chance of getting a disease sometime in one's lifetime. A half century ago, this was determined by evidence that a person's relatives had the disease or that a person showed alterations from simple blood tests or had other physical traits related to a disease. Today, the gene sequencing, as well as sophisticated blood tests, and advanced radiological exams, are often used. Combined, these have proven much more accurate in predicting predispositions than the original tests; however, the genetic tests are still not that accurate. First, not all genes involved in causing most diseases are known; second, the effect of the known polymorphisms are not always understood; third, not all the polymorphisms have been identified; fourth, the gene sequencing, especially of whole genomes, is not that accurate; and fifth, the actions of the epigenetic regulation of the disease related genes are not fully understood.

Currently, the known single nucleotide polymorphisms (SNPs) or other mutations in genes and abnormal gene functions (e.g., enzyme activities), that are currently known to play a role in a polygenic disease (caused by multiple genes), generally can only accurately predict a 10–20% chance of getting a disease in healthy patients. There is an approximately 20–40% accurate predictability in patients with symptoms or strong inheritance history. In contrast, with monogenic diseases with identified defects in the single causal gene involved, an accurate predictability is close to 100%. Similarly, in some instances, e.g., abnormal drug metabolism, when the enzyme gene is shown to be mutated, a range of the 80–100% range in predictability is achieved. In the future, the effects of epigenetic processes, i.e., alterations of gene expression by acetylation, methylation of the histones and DNA, etc., will also be used to enhance the accuracy in predicting predisposition. This entails simply measuring the RNA and protein expression of the genes of interest by a technique called "exon transcription analyses."

G.   Creating Individual Traits by Extremes in the Environment: Smoking, Radiation, etc.

It should be mentioned that the rate of both DNA (base) mutations and epigenetic changes can occur at an enhanced rate when an individual is exposed to certain factors in the environment, such as sunlight, temperature, chemical pollutant exposure (smoking, oxidants, and toxins), infectious agents, radiation, and dietary foods. Figure 8.2 outlines some recent data on the effects of smoking on incidence of lung cancer and the involved genomic mutations. A long-term smoking habit has been shown to create 23,000 additional DNA mutations in the smoker's lung tissue, not found in non-smokers. It has been calculated that

Figure 8.2

Effects of Tobacco Exposure on Small-Cell Lung Cancer Genome

Cigarette, Cigar, and Pipe Smoking
↓

- 60 chemicals that bind & mutate DNA – base attachment.

- Lung cancer develops, on average, after 365,000 cigarettes or 18,000 packs ($126,000 at $7/pack in 2012).

- 1 million new lung cancer patients each year worldwide.

  200,000 die each year in USA.   >90% are smokers.

⇓

The parallel sequencing of small cell carcinoma cell line (tobacco induced) compared to normal lung epithelial cell line, revealed:

- 23,000 DNA base mutations including 65 deletions, 334 copy number repeats, and 58 rearrangements.

- Inhibited repair of tumor suppressor genes and DNA.

- Estimated 1 DNA Mutation occurs for every 15 cigarettes.

Data taken from Pleasance et al, 2010

smoking enhances the mutation rate in the lung and other tissues 100 fold. The effects on epigenetic processes are not known, but they are suspected of being even greater. Such environmental factors can have a major effect on creating the individual, e.g., markedly enhancing disease incidence such as cancers, lung diseases, etc.

H.   Transgenerational Epigenetic Changes: Inheriting Epigenetic Changes

It is a bit shocking that Dr. Skinner and colleagues at the University of Texas at Austin and Dr. Rissman's laboratory at the University of Virginia have recently reported evidence in lab animals that environmental agents and stress that alter the epigenetics can have long-lasting effects – affecting generations in the future. There is evidence that a similar inheritance occurs in humans. This affect has been termed "transgenerational epigenetic changes." This makes sense, as once gene activity has been altered, i.e., epigenetic mechanisms have reset (genetic imprinting), the reversal of such changes may require a long time, even beyond the lifetime of an individual. However, proof that these observations are not due to permanent DNA changes, warrants more study.

I.   Novel Actions of Epigenetics on the Physiology, Mental Disorders, and Disease Predisposition of Future Generations

Scientists at the Heidelberg University reported in 2014 that the epigenetic DNA methylation and histone acetylation in the brain decreased in aged lab animals. Scientists now believe this decrease hinders neuron connections and stem cell regeneration resulting in the loss of neurons and reduced mental capacities. How this operates at the genetic/cellular levels is not understood. Evidence of a similar reduction in epigenetic activities resulted in decreased gene expression in animals with Alzheimer's-like conditions and with autopsies of

Alzheimer's patients. For example, transgenic mice bred with enhanced DNA demethylation (which activates gene expression) displayed much lower senility and increased memory functions as they aged. The genetic/epigenetic processes involving jumping genes (transposons) in neurons and adult stem cells, occurring as an embryo and adulthood, also appear to result in the unique (different) personalities, predisposition to mental diseases, and in learning. Recent studies suggest that these jumping gene sequences in the brain play a role in learning and helping an organism to adapt to its environment. It has been speculated that defects in these processes could also result in "abnormalities" in the brain causing mental diseases and mental limitations as they do in other organs. The scary possibility in these processes is that they appear to be inherited. Thus, no two humans will ever be exactly alike, not even identical twins. As we age, this individualism further increases due to the never ending epigenetic regulation which may even reach into future generations.

J.   Conclusions

This chapter dealt with the factors which create the individual human, even within ethnic populations and family members. These factors include the following:

• inheritance of unique genes from the parents;

• DNA (chromosomal) exchange, which mixes the unique genes of the mother and father, and the chromosomal distribution, occurring during sperm and egg production. This redistribution of the unique genes of the mother and father can create millions to billions of variations;

• add to this the selection of which sperm and egg to fertilize

• epigenetic regulation of gene expression in undifferentiated and differentiating cells, beginning when the embryonic cells differentiate. The extent of inheritance of the epigenetic patterns/processes is not fully understood. The variations and resulting possible outcomes are limitless.

Overall, scientists think that the reason our bodies have developed these chemical modifications for transcriptional regulation of genes, or have not eliminated the viral vestiges (jumping genes or transposons), is that they give us a better chance of survival by helping our genome to change and adapt to environmental demands.

The well-documented processes involved in germ cell (sperm and egg) formation (meiosis) and sperm selection, create unlimited genetic diversity in the individual, especially since it involves exchanges of unique parental genes. After birth, the random, natural errors in DNA replication, which begin at fertilization, as well as the induced environmental damage to the DNA, once created in germ cells, generally remain permanent in the genome. These newly created genetic mutations, occurring during a person's lifetime, contribute only slightly to this individual diversity, since these changes are few in number. In contrast, the accumulated polymorphisms in our genes, inherited from our parents and ancestors, and accumulated over thousands of generations, create unique genes that play a major role in our individualism. They create the unique genes we inherit. It is now commonly accepted that another dominant process in creating the individual involves epigenetic changes. As described above, and outlined Table 8.4 and in figure 8.3, epigenetics involves the differential regulation of gene expression by:

• determination of which of the maternal or paternal genes (alleles) will be expressed in the offspring (called genetic imprinting);

- chemical modifications (e.g., methylation) of the DNA bases and the regulatory proteins (histones and transcription factors) occurring throughout life;

- the regulation by micro (small) and long non-coding RNAs (ncRNAs);

- actions of transposons and retrotransposons; and finally

- variable levels and activities of the ncRNAs, transcription factors, and growth factors/cytokines add to this variability.

These are the primary processes involved not only in cell differentiation, but also in creating unique offspring and differences between siblings, i.e. individualism. It needs to be mentioned that there is an important connection between genetics (inherited genes and their polymorphisms) and epigenetics (gene regulation). There obviously exists the possibility for a regulation of regulatory genes. For example, some inherited polymorphisms are known to occur in epigenetic functioning genes (coding for microRNAs, lncRNAs, histone acetylases/deacetylases, etc.) which, in turn, can modulate the expression of a multitude of protein coding genes. Figure 8.3 gives an overview of the outcomes of epigenetic processes.

Currently, it is the pattern or specific single nucleotide changes (SNPs) that are usually used to predict disease susceptibility/predisposition. Most of these add only modest increases in predispositions because they involve only one or two of the many genes related to the development of a multigene based disease. These mutations often do not eliminate a gene function, as they only alter the activity of the gene.

With identical inherited patterns of polymorphisms and genes in identical twins, it is the unique epigenetic changes that are the major cause of the

Figure 8.3

Outcomes of Epigenetic Processes

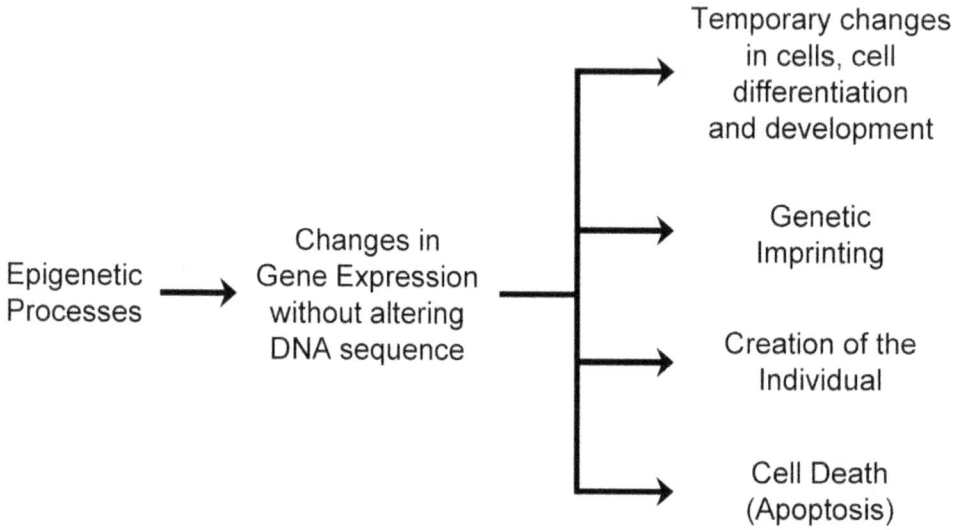

Epigenetic Processes → Changes in Gene Expression without altering DNA sequence →

- Temporary changes in cells, cell differentiation and development
- Genetic Imprinting
- Creation of the Individual
- Cell Death (Apoptosis)

(Thomas C. Spelsberg Ph.D., 2013)

differences that occur with aging in identical twins. During their lifetimes, identical twins will generate a few differential genetic (DNA) mutations that are minor compared to the more significant differences in their epigenetic (non-DNA) regulatory patterns. Thus, identical twins, starting with an identical genome, gradually become more different from each other as they develop *in utero* and age as adults. We now know that epigenetic processes, which are affected by differing environmental influences, are the basis for the differences between identical twins as they age. This explains their differences in appearances, fingerprints, metabolism, personality, and disease predisposition. Thus, Mother Nature's goal of "survival of the species" is answered by creating variations in each individual.

In summary, in addition to the well known inheritance of unique patterns of unique genes, epigenetic processes are believed to also be a major player in creating unique individuals, both physiologically (metabolically) and psychologically. Scientists are investigating the epigenetic processes, including how each one operates and which signaling pathways (gene functions) are altered. They are also investigating how stress and lifestyle alter these processes. Recently, scientists have discovered that select epigenetic processes can be long lasting and possibly maintained over several generations. So, what a great grandparent does (drugs, cigarette smoking, radiation exposure, etc.) may affect their great grandchildren. Maccani and coworkers at the University of Texas, Austin, recently reported that children of smokers had altered DNA methylation patterns (epigenetic regulation), including on genes related to diseases. This is, to say the least, a bit scary.

Scientists now know that much of the human genome is dedicated to epigenetic regulation via the microRNAs, the long non-coding RNAs and transposons (jumping genes). Scientists are now discovering that epigenetic regulation plays a major role in creating the individual. We can conclude that in addition to unique gene inheritance, the unique changes in the epigenetic regulation over time in individuals with millions of possible variations, create the differences in appearance, metabolism, moods, and personalities, disease susceptibility, and immune rejection of foreign tissues. One might envision individualism as Mother Nature's means to help humans as well as all animals, plants, and insects, to adapt and survive. Unfortunately the phenomenon also can cause cells to "lose control" and transform into altered (diseased) states such as cancer and mental disease.

Chapter 9

Future Roles of Individualized (Personalized) Medicine

Definitions

genetic/genomic sequencing: the sequencing of the whole genomic DNA of an individual; this includes protein coding and RNA coding genes, as well as intron and regulatory domains.

individualized medicine: the new field of medicine regarding each individual as unique and requiring individualized diagnoses and treatments of diseases.

monogenic diseases: rare diseases caused by mutations/defects in one essential gene; inactivation of these genes cause debilitating diseases that are excellent candidates for cure by gene therapy.

polygenic diseases: all common genetic diseases (i.e., those not caused by virus or bacterial infections or single gene defect) that are predisposed/caused by several to several defective genes; these defects can be DNA base changes or epigenetic expression changes.

A.   Introduction and Overview

The term "individualized medicine" is becoming increasingly popular. It is based on the fact that, as described in the previous chapter, individuals within a population are genetically unique not only due to their inherited unique genes, but also to the ever changing epigenetic processes. Individualized (personalized) medicine has been applied for years through the testing for blood types, certain polymorphisms, presence of hormone receptors, cancer markers, levels of metabolites and hormones, and more. One of the best examples of this uniqueness is the extensive tissue/organ rejection among human organ transplants.

This chapter describes the new medical field of individualized medicine and the promises it offers for medicine. The previous chapter described how and why humans become genetically unique. The fact that we all look different, have different personalities, display tissue incompatibilities, and have different disease predispositions, supports this individualism, even within the same ethnic population and families. Patients diagnosed with the same disease often display different outcomes and respond differently to the same drugs. This is because patients often have different variants of a disease, varying drug metabolism, drug responses, etc. As outlined previously in table 8.1, there are genetic differences in ethnic traits (physical and metabolic) caused by the inheritance of unique patterns of unique genes that are generated after many generations. This is due to genetic drift. The epigenetic (gene regulatory) processes between individuals add to the differences between individuals. Studies by Baye et al (2009) (see Table 8.1) have shown that these differences in genes among different populations are relatively modest compared to differences between individuals within these populations (see table 8.1). More detailed studies within populations have shown that gene sequence differences between individuals within a population, which cause many of the observed differences in physical appearance, metabolism, disease predisposition, etc., are markedly greater than those between populations [See Barbujani, et al, (1997) and Lewontin (1972) in Chapter 8 references]. Thus, the differences in inheritance patterns in the germ cells, and the ongoing epigenetic changes which occur after fertilization of the egg and beyond, generate traits unique to each individual, even between siblings and identical twins.

A prime example of the power and influence of individual genetic traits is the tissue/organ rejections with transplants between individuals, even between parents and siblings. This organ rejection is a real problem since even partial donor/recipient matches are only found at one out of hundreds or thousands of individuals. Identical twins and close relatives are better (but not perfect) matches, revealing their closer genetic make-up. This immune response of organ recipients is very sensitive, as it detects a multitude of markers on the membranes of implanted organs. Examples of other unique characteristics of individuals include physical appearances, disease predisposition, drug metabolism, personalities, and metabolic pathways. Identical twins are genetically very close, beginning life with an identical genome. However, due to epigenetic changes in each individual which occurs throughout life, they too generate unique traits as they age.

Thus, the application of "individualized/personalized medicine" to modern health care is certainly a much more accurate approach since it should provide better diagnoses and therapies, including drug selection and doses. Due to the multitude of molecular genetic determinants which make humans and animals unique, scientists cannot even come close in predicting all the specific unique features of an individual. The use of laboratory tests has only partially helped in identifying differences between individuals. Overall, personalized medicine is in its infancy, but has already been helpful in the practice of medicine.

B.   Obstacles to Personalized Medicine and the Medical Genetic Profiling of Individuals

Major obstacles to personalized medicine relate to the medical genetic profiling of people, not only in the DNA/gene sequencing, but also in the epigenetic analyses involving the analyses of the levels of activity of genes. The latter is only now just being studied with the protein/enzyme/metabolomics analyses. The main stumbling block to applying personalized medicine is our lack of markers related to metabolic diseases needed to personalize each individual. Many challenges lie ahead in order to make the field more practical and effective. Once these challenges have been met, personalized medicine will markedly improve medical treatments and certainly change how medicine is practiced. The following describes some of these obstacles and challenges:

(1)   The Cost of Sequencing a Whole Genome and Analyses of Gene Expression

Genomic sequencing has been used to identify a portion of the disease predispositions as well as subclasses of diseases based on genetic differences of the DNA. In 2000, the first sequence of a full genome (i.e., The Human Genome Project) cost $3 billion and was not that accurate. Since 2000, the price has been dropping with faster, more accurate analyses, using better techniques and instrumentation. In 2011 the cost was approximately $10,000—$20,000, but scientists are now claiming a $1,000/genome sequencing for 2014 and beyond. The real cost now seems to be both the more detailed and accurate sequencing and the computer analyses of this sequence once it is obtained. Some scientists claim that even a $1,000 sequenced genome may cost $10,000 and possibly more to be fully analyzed, especially with the multitude of added genes of the junk DNA and the more involved computer analyses. The latter falls under the field of "Bioinformatics." The analyses of the gene expression of the thousands of active protein coding genes in our tissues (the exomes) are still in the developing stages and they are both time consuming and expensive. The detailed analyses of the non-coding RNA genes, e.g., those of the micro and long non-coding types, have only just begun.

(2)   Accuracy and Speed of Sequencing and Gene Expression Analyses

DNA sequencing is not an absolutely accurate technique. The techniques are improving and requiring fewer replicate analyses, but occasional errors in this sequencing can hamper progress. Thus, repeat sequencing is currently required. Further, it took 7 years or more to perform the first full genome analyses. Current generation sequencing technologies are more accurate and more rapid. Future ones should be even more accurate, and hopefully will require only a few days or even one day. Full understanding of the medical implications of these genomes, however, will require longer periods of time using bioinformatics. The analyses of gene expression/activity (epigenetic regulation) are usually fairly accurate, but often require much more effort and money.

(3)   The Complexity and Differences of the Genomes and their Functions

Our human genome is vast, having 6 billion (6 thousand million) base pairs per diploid cell. Since our chromosomes are represented as homologous pairs, one from your mother and one from your father, only half (or 3 billion base pairs), called the haploid number, is usually sequenced. There is the issue of the homologous genes (alleles) located in our chromosome pairs as to whether one or both are differentially expressed and whether one dominates in functional activity. These processes are generally defined under the term "genetic imprinting," and more broadly under epigenetics. Also, as discussed in Chapter 8, no two humans have identical genomes (i.e., DNA) with 95% of the differences represented as base pair sequence differences between any two humans. This value represents approximately 6 million single base sequence differences (polymorphisms) between any two human individual diploid genomes. It should be reminded that 5% of total genomic differences actually include insertions, deletions, repeat sequences, and copy number variants, most of which have not been readily identified. Figure 9.1 outlines the current procedures used to identify polymorphisms associated with diseases. With the new discoveries that 80–90% of the junk genome is transcriptionally active and involved in epigenetic regulation of the protein coding genes, the need for accuracy of the whole genome sequencing becomes even more critical. Lastly, the regulation of thousands of genes, whether coding for protein or just RNA, is obviously complex, as described below.

(4)   Detecting Differences in Gene Expression Due to Epigenetic Regulation

As discussed previously, the differential epigenetic regulation of gene activity (expression) is one of the dominant forces behind individual differences. To assess this activity, analyses of mRNA and protein levels and enzyme activities must be performed. The ENCODE project is attempting to accomplish this with hundreds of individuals. Whole cells, isolated from each individual, help identify individual metabolic pathways. Figure 9.2 outlines some of the procedures used to

Figure 9.1

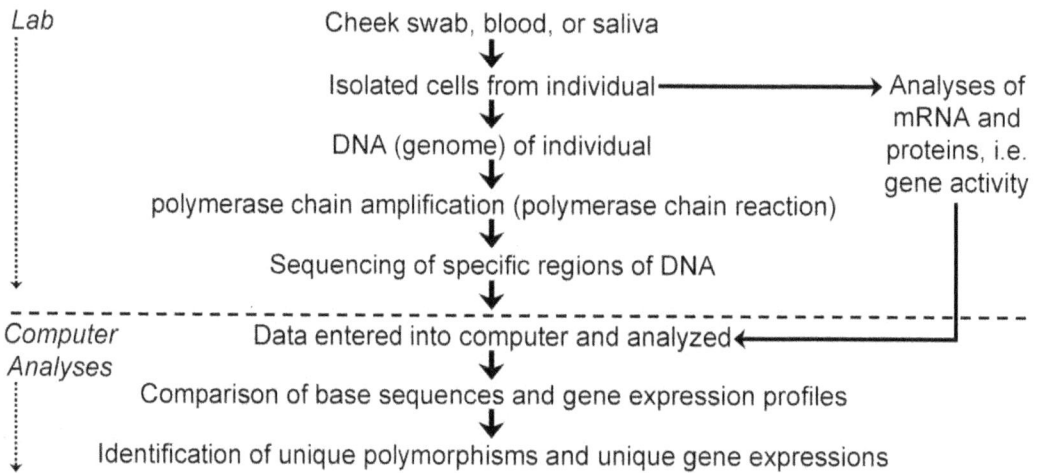

How Individual Genomic Analyses are Obtained

Lab

Cheek swab, blood, or saliva
↓
Isolated cells from individual ⟶ Analyses of
↓   mRNA and
DNA (genome) of individual   proteins, i.e.
↓   gene activity
polymerase chain amplification (polymerase chain reaction)
↓
Sequencing of specific regions of DNA
↓

Computer   Data entered into computer and analyzed ⟵
Analyses   ↓
Comparison of base sequences and gene expression profiles
↓
Identification of unique polymorphisms and unique gene expressions

(Thomas C. Spelsberg Ph.D., 2011)

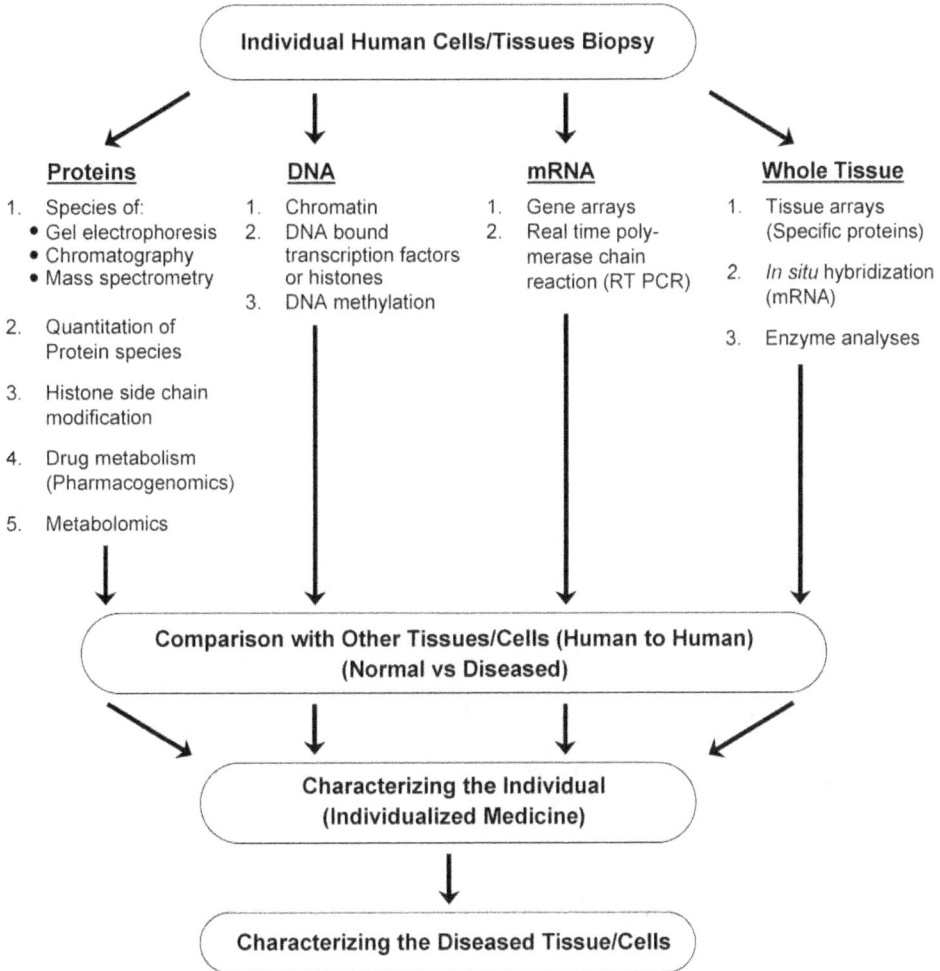

Figure 9.2

What's Involved in the Epigenic Analyses of Individuals

Individual Human Cells/Tissues Biopsy

Proteins
1. Species of:
   • Gel electrophoresis
   • Chromatography
   • Mass spectrometry
2. Quantitation of Protein species
3. Histone side chain modification
4. Drug metabolism (Pharmacogenomics)
5. Metabolomics

DNA
1. Chromatin
2. DNA bound transcription factors or histones
3. DNA methylation

mRNA
1. Gene arrays
2. Real time polymerase chain reaction (RT PCR)

Whole Tissue
1. Tissue arrays (Specific proteins)
2. *In situ* hybridization (mRNA)
3. Enzyme analyses

Comparison with Other Tissues/Cells (Human to Human) (Normal vs Diseased)

Characterizing the Individual (Individualized Medicine)

Characterizing the Diseased Tissue/Cells

(Thomas C. Spelsberg Ph.D., 2013)

characterize this unique gene regulation at the protein and RNA levels. While major technology development has enriched this area, attempts to interpret both the thousands of different protein and RNA molecular species and their "activities" (e.g., enzymes, growth factors, cytokines), as well as their interactions with other proteins, remain challenging even with today's technology. Studies of unique drug metabolism among individuals are pioneering this area under the auspices of pharmacogenomics. Pioneers in this field, such as Weinshilboum and colleagues at the Mayo Clinic, are designing ways to readily characterize the drug metabolic patterns of individuals. In addition, the identification of the select proteins/mRNAs that are unique to each disease (i.e., disease markers) can simplify the process and make this aspect of individualized medicine more practical.

(5)   Lack of Knowledge of Disease-related Protein Coding and Non-protein Coding Gene Domains

There remains the major challenge that many genes, whose altered expression or DNA mutation cause diseases, have yet to be identified. The non-protein coding gene domains that produce gene regulatory RNA molecules have also been implicated in human diseases. These represent the transposons/ retrotransposons, micro small RNA, and long non-coding RNA genes, all of which are only recently being assigned gene regulatory functions (see Chapter 8). The patterns of differential gene expression for hormone receptors, signaling molecules, enzymes, and others, are already serving as markers for specific diseases.

(6)   The Complexity of Polygenic Diseases

Most human diseases are caused by the alteration of several to many genes, i.e., they are "polygenic" diseases, as opposed to "monogenic" diseases that are caused by one defective gene (discussed in Chapter 10). A major obstacle in using genetic profiling of human diseases is the fact that many, if not most, of the genes involved in causing diseases have yet to be identified. Further, there is evidence that several different combinations of these genes cause the same general disease, but different subclasses (variants) of the same disease. As described in Chapter 8, this explains why using selected genes as markers for diseases usually only predicts a low percentage among the total population. Genome wide sequence studies in 2012 indicate that only a fraction, e.g., 10–20%, of the genes involved in causing a disease, are known.

Currently, scientists can accurately predict the future disease occurrence in only 10–25% of patients. In patients with a family history of the disease, there is a 25% prediction accuracy of that disease. It is much higher in patients with disease symptoms. However, in patients without symptoms, there is only a 10% or less prediction in the patient population as a whole using genetic analyses alone. In contrast, single gene disease predictions can reach 100%. In any case, the gene markers that are known are still assisting the physician to better characterize and predict the predisposition of a human disease. To better predict disease predisposition in the future, a multitude of patients with each disease needs to be analyzed to determine the full cadre of genes and the DNA and epigenetic changes which are involved in that disease. These data can then be correlated with disease incidence, subcategories of diseases, and disease outcomes.

(7)   The Need to Incorporate the Complete Clinical, Racial, Diet, and Stress Factors of a Patient

The environment and life style play a role in predisposition and disease incidence.

(8)   Our Livers and Our Gut Microbiome Can Create Unique Drug Responses

For many decades, physicians have understood that individuals and members of different ethnic populations respond differently to the same drug or doses of the same drug. Many of these individual drug effects have been assigned to specific drug metabolism enzymes in the liver, giving rise to the field of pharmacogenomics. More recently scientists are finding that certain gut microbe populations can affect (inactivate) the actions of certain drugs, and alter their effectiveness. Thus, the gut microbiome, partially unique to each human, can, in part, create a unique individual drug metabolism, thus making each of us more unique. This phenomenon makes predicting drug responses more difficult. It should be mentioned that when scientists assess the drug metabolites in the blood, the metabolism by gut microbes is included in this measurement, since these metabolites represent a summation of liver and microbe metabolism. As described in Chapter 6, our microbiome can affect our health and mental disposition, as well as our metabolism (including drug metabolism).

(9)   Obtaining and Handling the Genetic Data - Sequencing and Bioinformatics

Even though much progress has been made, research investigators are still plagued by: 1) inconsistencies in DNA sequencing results; 2) this is compounded by a lack of the "best" reference sequence. In short, what is not known is "which is the normal and which is the abnormal genome sequence;" 3) different commercial kits give different results; 4) the question, "which of the identified variances in the DNA sequence cause disease?" remains a major obstacle; and finally 5) all of the analyses require storage as well as comparative analyses of biological tissues of both healthy and diseased individuals by computers. The creation of "biobanks" of human tissues requires a major effort and funding, as there are vast amounts of information to be obtained, stored, and analyzed. These are costly endeavors under the auspices of "bioinformatics" which will be best achieved with coordinated efforts of many institutions and government support.

(10)   Ethical and Legal Issues

Finally, ethical and legal concerns have arisen as a result of genetic profiling and personalized medicine. There is the issue of close family relatives who could have many of the same disease predispositions as the patient under study. Is the physician obligated to inform them for the sake of their health without the patient's permission? What about using people's genetic profiles for disease-gene identification/correlation studies? Then there are concerns about having such knowledge in the hands of insurance companies, employers, etc. With the expected advances in genetic profiling (DNA, RNA, and protein), one negative aspect to be considered is that a more accurate prediction of a patient's future health would benefit insurance companies and employers which could then select to whom the insurance would be granted, or which diseases would be excluded from the insurance policy, or whom to hire.

C.   The Future: Hope, Promise, and Immediate Progress

One should not be depressed over the obstacles listed above because rapid advances are being made in the basic sciences and medicine. The fields of personalized medicine, pharmacogenomics, molecular biology, ancestry, anthropology, medicine, and bioinformatics have been reenergized by genomic analyses and more recently by epigenetic analyses. Advances have also occurred in engineering and computer technologies regarding genome and epigenome analyses. New opportunities are now arising since "predispositions" to diseases are now becoming available with expanded and improved genomic, epigenetic, and medical laboratory analyses. Patients should receive more focused and accurate checkups. Progress in the genetic analyses for disease predispositions, in the discovery of the genetic bases of diseases, as well as in the identification and defining subclasses of diseases, are in practice today and are leading to improved therapy. These discoveries are also leading to new therapeutic drugs, as well as the appropriate selection of drugs, and the most appropriate dosage to use with each individual. New genes related to diseases and their polymorphisms are being identified. New drugs targeting the functions of identified disease related genes are being developed. Unique therapies are also now being developed for each subclass of a disease in each individual. All humanity should benefit from any progress that is made in individualized medicine.

D.   Conclusions

Personalized medicine is already in practice today with the analyses of the family history, physical symptoms, blood composition, gene polymorphisms, and related disease indicators. Gene sequencing and epigenetic analyses (gene expression of RNA and protein levels) have further identified the uniqueness of the individual and that one size does not fit all. First, each individual inherits a unique pattern of genes from the sperm and egg formation and fertilization. Constant changes in gene expression patterns (epigenetics), described in the previous chapter, begin to occur in individuals immediately after the egg/sperm fertilization. The unique genetic inheritance and epigenetic regulation of gene expression creates the individual, as well as the need for individualized medicine within all populations. This unique genetic inheritance and epigenetic regulation are the foundations of the new individualized medicine. The latter has been recognized by the modern medical field as being much more important in medical diagnoses and treatments than just concerns over the immune system and organ rejections. Why the recognition of this need in the medical field has occurred only now? It is because we now have better understanding of- and tools to analyze- individual genetic and physiological attributes. In short, we can now better assess the individual's uniqueness.

The creation of each of us as individuals, largely by the differential genetic inheritance and subsequent epigenetic regulation of gene expression, are explaining the new field of Individualized (Personalized) Medicine, whereby we now realize that each individual in a population is significantly unique, both in genetic makeup and in epigenetic processes (physiology). This uniqueness includes their drug metabolism, immune compatibility, resistance to diseases, the predisposition as to the specific subclass of a disease, personality, and disposition.

It should be reminded that the individual exposure to environmental hazards, such as smoking or working around toxic substances and radiation, markedly increases the rate of genomic change (i.e., mutations of the DNA and probably epigenetic regulation) in individuals (see tables 8.2 and 8.3). As a result, an increase in specific disease incidence has been identified in those individuals exposed to hazardous environmental pollutants.

The identification of the full complement of disease causing genes combined with their DNA sequencing and the gene expression (epigenetics) analyses will help define who we are, with whom we are more compatible in organ transplants, our disease predisposition, and which drugs will or will not be most effective for each of us. The current analysis of an individual's unique genetic makeup, i.e., the pattern of gene expression and gene sequences, currently has the power to roughly predict one's health. In the future we will hopefully better predict one's health and have drugs to treat these diseases or modulate cellular processes, using inhibitors/activators of histone deacetylases and DNA methylases, etc. Improved genomic analyses should help identify disease causing genes and epigenetic processes in individuals. Lastly, the development of new drugs to modulate the epigenetic processes will open new opportunities for therapies for diseases, including mental diseases, as well as tissue regeneration.

The privacy issue is a major concern in personalized medicine. Related issues such as who is the true biological father, insurance companies' acceptance of clients, employer hiring selection, and which family members need to know about disease susceptibility, or even genetic relationships, are but a few. One wonders whether future genetic technology would lead us to a new order of genetic profiling similar to racial or religious profiling. It is not difficult for one to foresee a multitude of legal actions and laws over privacy, hiring, insurance, genetic profiling, and genetic bias. One might even envision that some individuals will want to select their mates for marriage or select their political leaders based on their genetic profile. In any case, let's not forget the immediate advantages of personalized medicine which offers:

- early detection of diseases;
- an improved prediction of predisposition;
- more efficient and more effective medical care;
- a better, more effective use of drugs with which to treat diseases; and ultimately,
- better health and longer living for humans and mammals.

Section IV

Curing Genetic Diseases – Gene Therapy

Chapter 10

Curing Genetic Diseases – Gene Therapy

Definitions

adenovirus: a non-enveloped virus containing double-stranded DNA and infecting mammals and birds, causing gastroenteritis and respiratory infections (colds, pneumonia). Efficient in infecting many cell types. Used here to carry large pieces of DNA into dividing cells and tissues for gene therapy.

adeno-associated viruses: similar to adenoviruses, but able to infect a variety of dividing cell types with little immune rejection, but can only carry small pieces of DNA.

gene delivery: the delivery of genes to cells/embryos using detergents, electrical fields, nano particles and viral particles.

retroviruses: viruses comprised of single-strand RNA animal viruses encoding a reverse transcriptase to produce DNA which then is inserted into host cell genome. Used to carry genes into non-dividing cells and tissues.

A.   <u>Introduction</u>

    (1)   <u>Background/History</u>

Gene therapy is a well known, evolving field of medicine that shows marked promise in curing devastating single gene diseases and selected multigene diseases. This chapter briefly describes this field, its history, uses, successes, and promises. For further reading on this topic, see the "References for Further Reading" section for this chapter at the end of this book and the internet. Gene therapy is usually applied to rare but severe diseases caused by defects (mutations) in a single gene, which displays loss or abnormal expression and function of this gene. The resulting gene deficiency or overexpression usually causes severe diseases. Its goal is to replace the defective gene and/or its regulatory neighboring regions. This therapy is of little use for more common diseases that are caused by multi-gene malfunctions, but there are exceptions. One exception could be the insertion/activation of a single tumor suppressor gene into cancer cells, a disease normally caused by many altered genes, to block cell proliferation and cancer growth.

On an historical perspective, interest in using genes for therapeutic applications arose in the late 1980s and flourished in the 1990s with one of the first applications to inhibit cancer growth by scientists such as Dr. French Anderson. The basic technique involves inserting a functioning "good" gene into a host cell to replace the defective, disease causing gene. Although flourishing in the 1990s, the field came under criticism in 1999 due to the death of an 18 year old patient, Jesse Gelsinger, who died by gene therapy for a non-fatal liver disease. Many trials were subsequently halted and some closed down. The field resurfaced anyway in the early 2000s largely due to pressures of parents seeking help/cures for their children who had these devastating genetic diseases causing blindness, physical deformities (e.g., dwarfism), defective immune systems (bubble children), intellectual disabilities, etc. Even though a second death due to gene therapy occurred in 2007, the field has still progressed. It is often the only real cure, or at least effective therapy, for most of these debilitating diseases of single gene defects. In the early 2000s, scientists reported successes in gene therapy in children with severe combined immunodeficiency syndrome (SCIDS). An example is Katlyn Demerchant of Canada who was freed from her bubble chamber at 5 years old, where she had lived her entire life. She was afraid and amazed at being outside her bubble and her home for the first time in her life, feeling the breeze and touching the grass, trees, other everyday items, including fellow humans.

Thus, gene therapy has been revitalized largely due to the severity of these single gene defective diseases and the ability of gene therapy to cure these diseases. Such therapies are allowing people to live long lives and have families. The concern now is that these achievements allow defective genes to be more readily passed on to future generations, avoiding Mother Nature's plan of "survival of the fittest." It is of interest to note that in 2014 Germany will sell the first commercial gene therapy kits for therapy of an inherited lipid disorder.

(2)   Current Challenges

Today, over 30 million Americans live with single gene diseases, both acute (deadly) and chronic (lifetime) forms. About 100 of these genetic abnormalities are more prominent. Many physical and metabolic abnormalities are caused by a single abnormal gene, resulting in the deficit or excess of one enzyme/protein or its function. These diseases are often devastating and involve dwarfism, chronic sickness/weakness, intellectual disabilities, blindness, organ failure, early death or life in a bubble chamber with no immune system, and many more. These individuals cannot obtain medical coverage and their medical bills are prohibitive. Since these diseases are inherited genetic diseases, physicians are at a dilemma as to how much to tell the immediate/distant family members, or even recommending gene therapy, due to the possible negative outcomes. However, the addition of one good normal gene to the patient with a defective gene, usually corrects the disease or at least reduces the symptoms. With the newly improved developed viral vectors and other delivery systems, many children with a variety of diseases are now being helped, if not "cured," of their diseases. One problem is the cost and another is "who pays." It is important to note that to eliminate a genetic disease from a family inheritance, the fertilized egg or the germ cells would have to be corrected via gene therapy. This aspect is further discussed at the end of this chapter.

B.   Examples of Current Advances and Activities

Since there are a multitude of gene therapy trials ongoing worldwide for a myriad of diseases, only listings of these trials are feasible in this chapter. These are presented as tables since full descriptions are beyond the scope of this book. The obstacles and selected advances in gene therapy studies are described below. Table 10.1 outlines all the gene therapy clinical trials by the phase of the trial and the worldwide geographical distribution of the trials. Table 10.2 provides a summary update, as of 2011, of documented gene therapy trials with known clinical outcomes. Table 10.3 lists many of the types of gene defects currently being corrected by the gene therapy trials. Table 10.4 lists the diseases currently undergoing gene therapy studies world wide according to the various organs and tissues of the body. Table 10.5 lists some of the commercial companies with gene therapies in clinical development. The following section will highlight a few of these clinical trials.

To give a brief overview of more recent advances, in 2008, an 8 year old boy, Corey Haas, was one of the first to be markedly helped by gene therapy for an incurable hereditary blindness. Blindness disorders, such as Leber's congenital amaurosis (an inherited blindness disease), have experienced the biggest success because the mitochondrial gene causing this disease was identified (see table 10.2). These gene therapies prevented blindness in 28 out of 30 patients. Gene therapies for immune disorders (i.e., immune deficiencies) soon followed, resulting, by 2011, in 86 patients worldwide being cured or helped (see table 10.2). All patients receiving therapy were cured by adding a functional (normal) gene to blood stem cells which differentiate into immune cells. These stem cells multiplied by the millions and differentiated into immune cells to restore normal immunity.

Scientists at the Cornell-Weill Medical College have had positive outcomes from gene therapy for beta-thalassemia and sickle cell disease by inserting the globin gene into bone marrow cells. Scientists at MIT are using antibodies and structurally altered proteins, both of which bind and inhibit certain growth promoting receptors (EGFR/HER-3, or HER-2), to inhibit cancer growth. Scientists at Fox Chase Cancer Center are activating receptor genes involved in hormone resistance and others are using drugs to directly block hormone receptors. Scientists at the University of California - San Francisco, using animal models with human related congenital deafness, have restored the hearing by injecting a viral-gene construct directly into the inner ear tissue. This therapy permanently restored

Table 10.1

A. Gene Therapy Trials Currently (2011) Active World Wide

Phase	Gene Therapy Clinical Trials	
	Number	% of Total
Phase I	1076	60.2
Phase I/II	333	18.6
Phase II	194	16.5
Phase II/III	16	0.9
Phase III	63	3.5
Phase IV	2	0.1
Single subject	2	0.1
Total	1786	~100

B. Geographical Distribution of Clinical Trials of 2011

Country	Number	% of Total
USA	1143	64
UK	201	11.3
Germany	81	4.5
Switzerland	50	2.8
France	49	2.7
Australia	29	1.6
Netherlands	29	1.6
Belgium	25	1.4
China	23	1.3
Canada	22	1.2
Italy	21	1.2
All Other	112	6.4
TOTAL	1786	100

Taken from J. of Gene Medicine - Online:
http://www.wiley.com/legacy/wileychi/genmed/clinical

Table 10.2
Outcomes of Gene Therapy 2000 - 2011

Disorder	Resulting Disease	Patients Benefiting
I. Gene Therapy for Genetic Disease		
• X-SCID	Immunodeficiency	17of 20
• ADA-SCID	Immunodeficiency	26 of 37
• Adrenoleukodystrophy	Neurologic	2 of 4
• Duchenne muscular dystrophy	Muscle loss	19 of 19
• Leber's congenital amaurosis	Blindness	28 of 30
• Wiskott-aldrich syndrome	Immunodeficiency	8 of 10
• β-thalassemia	Hemoglobinopathy	1 of 1
• Hemophilia	Coagulation	6 of 6
II. Gene Therapy for Degenerative Disease		
• Heart failure	Heart	9 of 9
III. Gene Therapy for Cancer		
• β cell leukemia and lymphoma	Blood cancer	6 of 8
• Acute leukemia	Blood cancer	4 of 5
• Squamous cell carcinoma	Head and neck cancer	14 of 16
• Melanoma	Skin cancer	92%
• Metastatic solid tumors	Solid tumors	14 of 16

Taken from J. Kaiser, 2011, Gene Therapists Celebrate a Decade of Progress. Science 334:29-30; and L.W. Seymour & A.J. Thrasher, 2012, Gene Therapy Matures in the Clinic. Nature Biotech. 30:588-593.

Table 10.3

Types of Genes being Corrected by Gene Therapy Trials

Gene type	Gene Therapy Clinical Trials as of 2011	
	Number of Trials	% of all Trials
Adhesion molecule	10	0.6
Antigen	370	20.7
Antisense	13	0.7
Cell protection/Drug resistance	19	1.1
Cytokine	331	18.5
Deficiency	141	7.9
Growth factor	134	7.5
Marker	54	3
Oncogene regulator	12	0.7
Cancer virus	37	2.1
Porins, ion channels, transporters	12	0.7
Receptor	125	7
Replication inhibitor	77	4.3
siRNA	11	0.6
Cell destruction	148	8.3
Transcription factor	28	1.6
Tumor suppressor	152	8.5
Others	32	1.8
Unknown	52	2.9
Total	1786	100.00

Taken from J. of Gene Medicine - Online:
http://www.wiley.com/legacy/wileychi/genmed/clinical/

Table 10.4

Diseases Currently (2012) Undergoing Gene Therapy Clinical Trials

Organ/System

Brain
  Glioblastoma
  Huntington's

Bone
        Orthopedic Repair
        Osteoporosis
        Postmenopausal

Cancer
        Liver, GI, Skin, Connective
Tissue,
        Bone, Breast, Prostate, Brain,
        Retina

Diabetes

Eye
        Retinal Degeneration
        Cornea Glaucoma
        Daylight Blindness
        Ocular Disease
        Retinal Ganglion Cell

Pulmonary Hypertension
        (Heart to Lung)

Skin
        (Melanoma)

Spinal Muscular Dystrophy and Atrophy

Vascular (Blood Vessels)
        Atherosclerosis
        p53 Therapy

Hearing
        Cochlia, Inner Ear

Heart
        Ischemia, Angiogenesis
        Electrical Dysfunction

Hemophilia
        Chronic Granuloma
        Leukodystrophies
        Hemophilia

Immune System
        H.I.V., SCIDS (deficiency)

Inherited/Acquired Liver Diseases

Lysosomal Storage Diseases

Neurological
        Degenerative Diseases
        Peripheral Nerve Disease

Taken from J. of Gene Medicine - Online:
http://www.wiley.com/legacy/wileychi/genmed/clinical/

Table 10.5
Selected companies with gene therapies in clinical development as of 2012

Company	Product	Indication	Clinical status
uniQure	Alipogene (Glybera)	Lipoprotein lipase deficiency	Pending approval
	AMT-060	Hemophilia B	Phase ½
Advantagene (Auburndale, Massachusetts)	ProstAtak kinase	Prostate cancer	Phase 3
		Glioma	Phase 2
		Pancreatic cancer	Phase ½
GlaxoSmithKline (London)	Encoding adenosine deaminase (ADA)	ADA deficiency in severe combined immunodeficiency (SCID)	Phase 3
Vical (San Diego)	Allovectin	Melanoma	Phase 3
Applied Genetic Technologies (Alachua, Florida)	alpha-1 antitrypsin gene	Alpha-1 antitrypsin deficiency	Phase 2
Bluebird Bio	Lenti-D	Adrenoleukodystrophy	Phase 2
	Lentiglobin (human beta-globin gene)	Beta thalassemia	Phase 2
Celladon (San Diego)	Mydicar	Cardiomyopathy	Phase 2
Ceregene	Cere-120	Parkinson's disease	Phase 2
	Cere-110 (NGF)	Alzheimer's disease	Phase 2
Genzyme (Cambridge, Massachusetts)	AAV-hAADC-2 (the human aromatic l-amino acid decarboxylase gene)	Parkinson's disease	Phase 2
Oxford BioMedica	ProSavin	Parkinson's disease	Phase 2 (complete)
Shenzhen SiBiono GeneTech (Shenzen, China)	Gendicine (human P53)	Lung cancer	Phase 2

The US National Institutes of Health Clinicaltrials.gov website lists 2,965 gene therapy trials, of which 1,103 are listed as recruiting. The vast majority of these are being directed by academic investigators.

inner ear cell functions and hearing. Recently Pinyon and colleagues at the New South Wales University in Sydney, Australia, delivered the neurotrophin gene into inner ear cells of deaf Guinea Pigs. The auditory nerve regenerated and the hearing was restored in the pigs. Mendell and coworkers at the National Children's Hospital in Columbus, Ohio, used adenovirus constructs, to add the Follistatin gene to muscles of three patients with muscular dystrophy. This gene functions to activate muscle growth. This therapy restored much of the muscles that received the viral gene therapy. Lastly, scientists at UCLA are working on gene therapy models for mutated (inactivated) mitochondrial genes. These maternally inherited mitochondrial gene mutations cause severe muscular and neuronal diseases, Alzheimer's, cancer, and diabetes. "Mitochondrial replacement" therapies are also being tested with some successes in animal models with certain diseases.

New studies are ongoing to diminish/cure diseases, not only to insert new genes into cells/organs, but also to selectively induce or inhibit the expression of the host endogenous genes which cause diseases by being abnormally expressed. Using this approach on laboratory animals, scientists at Heidelberg University, Germany, enhanced the DNA demethylation enzyme activities (epigenetic actions) in the brains of animals to enhance host (endogenous) gene expression patterns. This treatment improved their memory, learning, and awareness. Such approaches are being considered for Alzheimer's and related disorders. Other studies in lab animals have applied gene therapy to enhance heart regeneration in adult cardiac stem cells (discussed in Chapter 12).

C.   Advances and Obstacles in the Delivery of a Gene to the Targeted Cells of the Diseased Patient

Adequate laboratory techniques to efficiently deliver genes to target cells have been a major obstacle in this field. Initial studies involved inserting genes into isolated cell populations by a variety of means such as lipofection (lipid droplets), electrophoresis (electrical stimulation), mild detergents, and viral vectors. By far, viral vectors attached to the gene of interest have proven most effective. Viral DNA or RNA are stripped of the genes involved in developing diseases and altered to prevent their capacity to replicate. The gene of interest is then inserted into this modified viral DNA (genome) along with any control segments (promoters) for regulating the activity of the gene. These DNA constructs are repackaged into viral particles which maintain the ability to infect specific cell types. Overall, the ideal vector for gene therapy needs to be readily available, safe (not generating an immune response), efficient (infecting many cells), and able to target specific cell types. Finally, the inserted gene needs to be functional in the targeted cells and inserted permanently into the host DNA. The viral vector of choice, depends on the disease to be treated, the size of DNA needed to be inserted, and the physician/scientist's decision based on the disease. The primary viral vectors used so far are the retroviruses (RNA based viruses), adenoviruses (DNA based viruses) and the adeno-associated viruses.

Retroviruses (e.g., lentivirus) have the advantage that they can infect and integrate into the host cell DNA of non-dividing cells. These are often used in studies of neurological disorders. Drs. Russell, Dispenzieri, and co-workers at the Mayo Clinic are currently making marked advances in safely using the altered measles virus (RNA based) and other related viruses for use in gene therapies in a variety of cell types in animals and humans. In one case, they treated a woman with final stages of myeloma cancer with high doses of a measles viral construct that inhibits a certain growth promoting receptor protein on the membranes of myeloma cancer cells. She has displayed a remarkable full recovery, at least at several months post-therapy as a result of this team's efforts.

Adenoviral vectors have the advantage of being able to infect many different cell types and to insert large pieces of DNA. However, they sometimes generate harmful, if not deadly, immune responses. In contrast, the adeno-associated viruses usually do not cause immune rejection, they have the ability to infect a wide variety of cell types, and can function either outside the chromosomes (as an independent piece of DNA) or as part chromosomal DNA of the target cell. However, they can only insert a small piece of DNA.

D.   Current Risks of Gene Therapy

Problems with gene therapy occasionally arise when the viral vector, used to insert genes into cells, causes unwanted results. These can be categorized into three effects:

(1)   Adverse Host Responses to the Viral Vectors or to the Newly Added Gene: An adverse immune response to gene therapy can be lethal or make one sick for extended periods. The transferred gene or its viral carrier could produce a protein which creates an immune response or can disrupt body functions. There may be an over-production or under-production of the protein produced by the injected gene caused by a lack of appropriate regulation. All of these potential hazards need to be tested beforehand.

(2)   Causing Cancer: On occasion, the transferred gene or its vector integrates into the patient's DNA and activates a cancer causing proto-oncogene or blocks an anticancer gene (tumor suppressor gene), either of which can encourage cancer. The new design of viral vectors has reduced the concern of activating

cancer enhancing genes. However, the concern of inactivating one or more of a cell's tumor suppressor gene remains a problem.

(3)   The Inactivation of a Host Gene by Virus: The virus used in the therapy can inactivate an essential gene for cell viability. This is generally not an issue, but has been documented in the past.

Even with these concerns, the genetic diseases are so devastating that the advantages of gene therapy have proven highly worthwhile. This is especially true with the development of new technological advances. It even has the potential to stop inherited diseases in families forever, when the technology can be applied to fertilized eggs at early stages.

E.   Ethical Considerations

As expected, there are ethical considerations regarding gene therapy. Some of these include:

(1)   Information: Whether or not to inform relatives of the genetic abnormality which could be in their genes (as carriers). In some patients the gene of concern may act in a recessive manner, i.e., not causing the disease, but can be passed on to the next generation who might develop an active disease.

(2)   Fighting Mother Nature: Fighting Mother Nature's "survival of the fittest" by curing genetic diseases in people, allows us to procreate in greater numbers, even when having the genetic disease. In this case, we can pass on the defect to many offspring in the following generations. Under normal scenario, these genetic disease carriers would not have offspring, which tends to eliminate/reduce the disease from a population, i.e., natural selection.

Note: Gene therapy is currently not performed on germ cells (sperm and egg). Although the patient may be cured of the disease and its symptoms, the genetic defects are often passed on to offspring via sperm or egg. Gene therapy of germ cells should eliminate the disease from the family forever, and help reduce the disease from the population. Alternatively, the fertilized eggs or early embryos could be tested for presence of the genetic defect and only the "healthy" egg "embryo" selected for birth.

(3)   Cost: There is a high cost for gene therapy, therefore, one has to ask, "Who gets the gene therapy treatment?" However, this therapy is markedly cheaper than the chronic treatment of the genetic disease's symptoms throughout the lifetime of the patient.

Section V

Regenerating our Organs: Regenerative Medicine

Chapter 11

Regenerative Medicine: The Power and Universality of the Human Stem Cell

Definitions

cytokines: see Growth Factors

embryonic stem cell (totipotent): totipotent or pluripotent stem cells in the embryo which can generate most (pluripotent), if not all (totipotent), cell types in the human body.

growth factors/cytokines (paracrine factors): proteins secreted by one cell to bind to membrane receptors of neighboring cells to regulate cell division and cell functions, including cell differentiation. Act as cell to cell communicators.

induced pluripotential stem cell: laboratory generated stem cells using 4 key regulatory genes inserted into mature differentiated (adult) cells which then cause the de-differentiation into a stem cell. Many cell types, e.g., the skin or bone marrow, can be used as a target for these 4 genes. These cells can then be differentiated into many cell types. They resemble embryonic stem cells. These cells allow regeneration of tissues in the same patients from whom the stem cells were generated, which eliminates rejection.

natural adult stem cell (multipotent): stem cells naturally occurring in adult tissues that are able to differentiate into several specific adult cell types of that tissue or organ.

paracrine factors: see growth factors

regenerative medicine: the medical field that uses stem cells to repair damaged or dead tissues or organs.

somatic stem cell: same as natural adult stem cell above. One of mitotically active, undifferentiated (i.e., uncommitted) somatic "stem" cells in most adult tissues that can replenish several different cell types, allowing natural tissue regeneration (e.g., skin repair).

A. Overview and History

Regenerative medicine is a relatively novel field of medicine that holds great promise for the repair of tissues and organs. This chapter deals with animal and human stem cells, which are the cells that can differentiate and replenish tissues, and includes descriptions of their origins, properties, and functions. For more details in this field, including its history, read "Stem Cell Research" by Joseph Panno (2010), and for a general overview read, "Stem Cells for Dummies" by Goldstein and Schneider (2010), under the "References for Further Reading" section for Chapter 11. Also, the internet searches are beneficial.

Many adult animals can regenerate parts of their bodies. Salamanders can regenerate limbs, retinas, and parts of the brain after surgical or accidental loss. Zebra fish can regenerate two-thirds of their hearts that have been cut away. Tadpoles can regenerate their tails. Flatworms (e.g., planaria) can completely regenerate themselves as whole organisms even after being cut into pieces. Amazingly, each piece regenerates a new individual worm. Many animals can regenerate their limbs as embryos. As discussed in Chapter 4, even adult humans can regenerate portions of their liver, skin, blood cells, and intestinal cells. Children, ages 12 years and younger, can regenerate the last one-fourth to one-half inch of their fingertips, while adults cannot do so. Children can also regenerate parts of their tissues much faster than older humans who lose much of this capacity. All of these regenerations are possible because these tissues/organs contain adult stem cells, and express the necessary growth factors to activate and direct stem cell growth and regeneration. When activated, the stem cells regenerate the appropriate cell types, tissue structures, and functions of the tissues in which they reside.

Regenerative medicine involves the use of the body's own adult stem cells, or those from another person or embryonic cells, to regenerate normal tissue to replace diseased or damaged tissues. Significant scientific/medical breakthroughs have occurred over the past 10—20 years, which open the possibility for us to regenerate many parts of the human body. It has been known for over a century that the fertilized egg will divide to produce several types of embryonic stem cells that continue to divide and differentiate into approximately 200 mature differentiated cell types. Scientists have been able to accomplish parts of this differentiation outside (in vitro) as well as inside (in vivo) living animals and humans.

Humans constantly undergo natural regeneration to repair damaged/worn out tissues, including dying aged cells. Humans endure, knowingly or unknowingly, the natural regeneration/repair of damaged skin, livers, hearts, pancreases, skeleton, kidneys, muscles, connective tissues, and nerves. A young person repairs much faster and better than an aged person, since young humans have greater numbers and more active stem cells. This is the period of "healing" from an injury. These repairs were finally identified as due to the presence of regenerating adult stem cells that reside in most, if not all, of the organs and tissues of our adult human and animal bodies. Stem cells, located in bone marrow, can circulate in the blood and lodge in damaged areas, partially differentiate, and repair many tissues. Stem cells require removal of scar tissue to regenerate new tissue.

In 1908 a histologist, Alexander Maksimov, found that certain bone marrow cells could differentiate into various blood cells. He termed these cells, "stem cells," referring to how a tree trunk/stem gives rise to many branches. It was not until the 1940s—50s and the atomic age that interest in such cells was resurrected because the need of healing humans from the damages of radiation. In the 1960s, John Gurdon showed that the cell nucleus from an adult frog would differentiate when placed in an unfertilized egg and result in a "cloned" frog. Dr. Wilmut and colleagues repeated this phenomenon with adult sheep in the 1990s. These studies demonstrated that cell differentiation was reversible. In 1998, Jim Thomson and colleagues at the University of Wisconsin-Madison were one of the first to culture embryonic stem cells and demonstrate their potential to differentiate into adult tissues in culture (in vitro). Using undifferentiated stem cells combined with select growth factors, hormones, cytokines, and vitamins (to help direct the differentiation), scientists are now able to reproduce many tissues of the body in laboratory cultures. Figure 11.1 outlines how these different classes of stem cells are created and used by the human body. Table 11.1 lists the types and characteristics of various stem cells. As outlined in table 11.2, a class of stem cells, called adult stem cells, has been found in bone, blood, brain, digestive tract, heart, pancreas, retina, muscle, cartilage, connective tissue, and skin. These partially committed (i.e., partially differentiated) stem cells can regenerate a limited number of cell types and parts of organs found in their tissue of origin. The regeneration of whole organs has yet to be achieved.

An important follow-up discovery demonstrated that the differentiation of these stem cells is guided by specific growth factors and cytokines produced by the remaining (surrounding) cells of each organ. These chemical signals encourage the stem cells to proliferate and determine the direction of the adult stem cell's differentiation. One of the first of these factors was isolated and characterized by Dr. Cohen (Vanderbilt) and Dr. Montalani (France), as epidermal

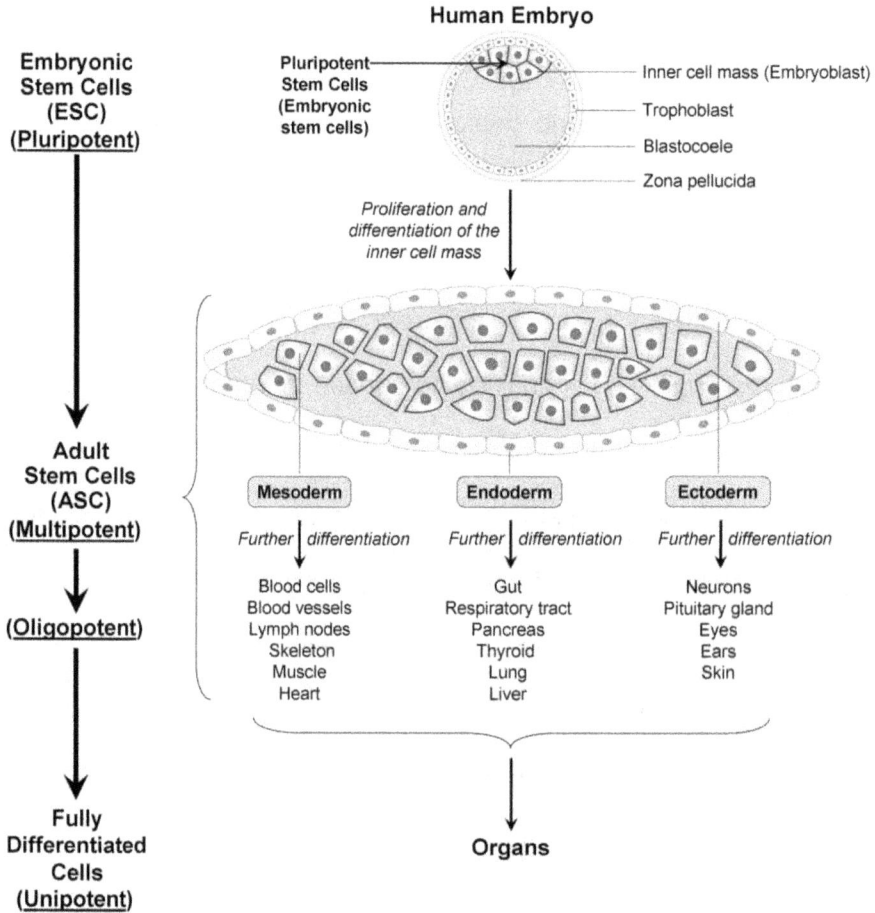

Figure 11.1

From Embryo to Adult Tissues (Role of Stem Cells)

Selected information taken from J. Panno, 2010.

Table 11.1

Classes of Human Stem Cells

TYPE	SOURCE	POTENTIAL
Totipotent cells from fertilized egg	Earliest embryo (1-16 cells)	Can create whole organisms and all 240 cell types
Pluripotent cells from human embryonic stem cells (ES Cells)	More mature embryo (5 day) (100 cells)	Can create most cell types (~110 types or more)
Multipotent cells from human embryonic germ cells (EG Cells) and adult tissues	Fetus (5-9 weeks) (Millions of cells) And adult tissues*	Partially differentiated; can only differentiate into a limited number of cell types (2-10)
Induced pluripotent stem cells (iPS cells) from adult stem cells treated with a cohort of transcription factors	Adult tissues stem cells with transcription factor over-expression	Can create most cell types usually without rejection, when the same individual is used as a source.
* Found in adult tissues to repair and replace body tissue when damaged.		

Table 11.2

Adult Organs with Adult Stem Cells

Adult Tissue/Organ	Characteristics
Bone marrow	Contains mesenchymal stem cells, that differentiate into cartilage and bone, and endothelial progenitor cells, that differentiate into blood vessels and cardiomyocytes. Hematopoietic stem cells that differentiate into red and white blood cells.
Brain	Brain stem cells differentiate into the three kinds of nervous tissue – astrocytes, oligodendro-cytes, and neurons, including some dopamine neurons.
Digestive system	These stem cells renew the epithelial lining of the gut. They are located in intestinal invaginations.
Heart	The heart stem cells reside in small clusters in the heart lining.
Pancreas	Neural stem cells can generate pancreatic β cells.
Skeletal muscle	Stem cells mediate muscle growth and proliferate in response to injury or exercise. They reside in muscle and bone marrow.
Skin	Skin stem cells repair and replace all types of skin cells. Skin stem cells are associated with the epithelial cells, epidermal cells, hair follicle cells, and the basal layer of the epidermis.
Retina	Retinal stem cells recently have been found in the pigment epithelial cells. They keep rods and cones healthy and can proliferate and regenerate the retina, lens, and neurons.

Table 11.2. Select data taken from: J. Panno (2010), "Stem Cell Research," Checkmark Books, 132 West 31st Street, New York, NY

growth factor (EGF). A major discovery was announced several years ago when Japanese scientists were able to de-differentiate mature cells into embryonic-like cells that can differentiate into many cell types. This was achieved by the insertion of several key regulatory genes into differentiated cells. The isolation of stem cells and their direct differentiation into the desired cell types represent the foundation of the new field of "regenerative medicine." This chapter describes the various "stem cells" used in regenerative medicine, the role of growth factors and cytokines in directing their differentiation, and the repair of many tissues due to injury or aging.

B.   Mother Nature's Primary (Totipotent/Pluripotent) Stem Cell: The Fertilized Egg and Embryonic Stem Cells

Most readers are aware that humans and all higher organisms begin life as a single cell fertilized egg. This cell is a totipotent or pluripotent stem cell, which divides again and again to eventually become a whole organism (see figure 11.1). In the case of humans, an end result is a baby with approximately 10^{13} cells (10 trillion) and 200 cell types. This scenario occurs in all living multicellular organisms. This biological process is termed the development or Ontogeny of an organism. This occurs in all living multicellular organisms, e.g. plants (from grass to redwood trees), insects, and animals, including humans, snakes, clams, fish, birds, fungi, etc. As outlined in figure 11.1, the process first involves the repeated cell divisions of the fertilized egg to create a population of embryonic stem cells. These cells continue to divide and differentiate to create cells with the accompanying changes in cell structures/shapes and functions due to cell differentiation. This process leads to tissues, organs, and eventually the development of the whole organism (e.g., frogs, worms, sheep, and other farm animals). This process of changing cell properties and functions is termed "cell differentiation" caused by the epigenetic regulation of gene expression. The embryonic cells are "programmed" by Mother Nature, as "totipotent" or "pluripotent" stem cells, to differentiate into all different cell types, including the roughly 200 types in humans and mammals. A lesser number of differentiated cell types are found in worms, jelly fish, and other less complex animals.

As outlined in figure 11.1, and discussed below, some partially differentiated stem cells (adult multipotent stem cells) continue to function in organs and mature tissues throughout our lifetimes to carry out limited repair/regeneration. For more than a century, scientists have been able to partially mimic this cell differentiation of embryonic cells using cell culture techniques in the laboratory. As mentioned earlier, scientists were eventually able to develop whole organisms, e.g., frogs, sheep, etc. from fertilized eggs and stem cells in a procedure known as "cloning." Examples of lab generated cell types from stem cells are listed in table 11.3.

C.   Natural (Multipotent) Adult Stem Cells and the Natural Tissue Regeneration in Our Bodies

Even as adults we are continuing to regenerate new tissue every minute of our lives. Every day over 200 billion (2×10^{11}) cells or 0.2 to 2% of our total number of human body cells, are destroyed and replenished in our bodies by adult stem cells. Red blood cells and skin cells are being replaced with fresh, undamaged cells at a rate of millions of cells per minute. The billions of cells living in our intestines are completely replaced every week. Even the total skeleton (bone) in our bodies is completely replaced every 7 to 10 years or so during our lifetime. Partial natural regeneration occurs in all organs, such as the brain and heart, but

Table 11.3

Names and Functions of Differentiated Cell Types which have been
Generated in the Laboratory from Stem Cells

Cell Name	Cell Type/Function
Adipocyte	Fat cells
Astrocyte	Brain cells that provide support to the neurons
Cardiomyocyte	Heart cells that form the heart
Chondrocyte	Cartilage cells (connective tissue)
dendritic cells	Cells of the immune system
endothelial cell	Blood vessel cells
hematopoietic cells	Blood cells
Keratinocyte	Hair and nail cells
mast cell	Connective tissue and blood vessel cells
Neurons	Brain, spinal cord, and peripheral nerve cells
Oligodendrocyte	Myelin-forming nerve cells
Osteoblast	Bone-forming cells
pancreatic islet cells	Insulin synthesizing cells
smooth muscle	Blood vessel and digestive tract cells

Table 11.3. Selected information taken from: J. Panno (2010)

only partial, never the whole organ. This astonishing regeneration in our bodies is due to the partially differentiated adult stem cells in our adult organs and tissues (see figure 11.1 and list in table 11.2). These natural adult stem cells, first discovered in the 1960s in bone marrow for blood cells, reside in all of our organs and tissues. They are partially differentiated, and thus limited, as per the cell type of that tissue/organ. Thus, these cells are classified as "multipotent" (not "totipotent") stem cells. Interestingly, adult stem cells from babies can divide up to 50 times while those from older adults can only divide 10—20 times, and there are fewer of them. Thus, our tissue regeneration (repair) slow as we age. I am sure many of us who have aged have become aware of this.

D.   Laboratory Studies of Natural Adult Stem Cells from Tissues and Organs

As outlined in figure 11.1 and mentioned above, natural adult stem cells represent the partially differentiated stem cells found in the tissues/organs of babies, children, and adults. These are derived from the early embryonic cells from which all of the body's differentiated cells are made. Although originating in the early embryo, the partially differentiated (i.e., multipotent) natural, adult stem cells remain in adult organs and tissues for a lifetime to carry out future tissue repair with the ability to replenish a limited number of cell types of that organ. These cells divide to replenish worn out dying cells when needed, and as multipotent cells, differentiate into a limited variety of cell types found in that organ. This ability obviously gave survival advantage to humans and other animals.

Historically, about a half century ago, two Canadian scientists, Drs. McCullock and Till, discovered adult stem cells. They discovered that many tissues in adult organisms harbor unique cells that are actively dividing "stem cells," and are able to differentiate into mature cell types found in the tissue in which they reside. However, it was in the 1990s and early 2000s that significant interest in adult stem cells arose, as indicated by books and research publications on the topic. As mentioned above, there was a breakthrough in 1998 when Dr. Thomson's labs at the University of Wisconsin, Madison, reported methods to isolate and grow embryonic stem cells and partially direct them to differentiate into certain cell types. This was followed by the isolation of natural adult stem cells by Dr. Verfaille (University of Minnesota) in the bone marrow and blood. Since 2006, significant discoveries have been made by isolating adult "stem" cells from tissues and organs in animal and humans. These "adult stem cells" can differentiate into many cell types found in the organ in which they reside. These cells are now classified as multi-potent (i.e., producing many) cell types, as opposed to the toti- or pluri-potent (i.e., producing all cell types). Since then, scientists have developed techniques to isolate endogenous adult stem cells from many organs by enriching these scarce cells from the large number of mature cells, using cell sorting machines.

To summarize, the embryonic stem cells, which can differentiate into all cell types of a human (e.g., approximately 200 different types), are termed "totipotent" or "pluripotent." In contrast, the "adult stem cells" in organs are termed "multipotent adult stem cells" because they can differentiate only into a limited number of cell types found in that organ. Adult stem cells that have been cultured in the lab and the cell types they have generated are listed in table 11.3. Scientists have elucidated a simplified developmental process in living organisms. As outlined in figure 11.1; the original pluripotent embryonic (stem) cell (fertilized egg) gives rise to "adult stem cells" which, in turn, give rise to the final, specialized, cells used by the infant (or any newborn animal) to survive.

E.   The Laboratory Generated "Induced Pluripotential Stem Cells"

Scientists are currently using cell culture and genetic technologies to reverse Mother Nature's natural processes. One of the most significant and major breakthroughs was reported in 2007 by Yamanaka and colleagues at the Kyoto University. They reported that the combined expression of four regulatory genes (transcription factors, termed Oct-4, Sox-2, Klf-4, and c-myc) in differentiated adult animal cells causes a "de-differentiation" into a totipotent/multipotent type of stem cell. Dr. Thomson and colleagues at the University of Wisconsin reported similar findings that year. As outlined in figure 11.2, these cells can then be re-directed to differentiate into many, if not all, differentiated cell types (Takahashi et al, 2007). This achievement was awarded the Nobel Prize to Dr. Yamanaka. These cells called "induced pluripotent stem cells" (iPS cells) and represent the preferred and major approach used in regenerative medicine studies today.

Later, in 2013, Mitalipov and colleagues created human iPS cells. Some applications of these iPS cells are listed in figure 11.2. The iPS cells do not appear to have the limitations of adult stem cells and are currently the cell type of choice for most stem cell studies. The iPS cells can be generated from cells of the same patient who requires new tissue.   This avoids tissue rejection by the immune system. Figure 11.2 outlines this process of inserting of several regulatory genes into fully differentiated adult cells to create these induced pluripotent stem cells (iPS cells). Problems with this technique in the past have been that only 10% of the target cells to be "induced" are actually de-differentiated into stem cells and the process can take months to achieve. However, scientists at the Weizman Institute of Science (Israel) have recently identified a protein, called Mbd3, which blocks the

Figure 11.2

Cell Types Differentiated from Embryonic and Adult (Organ) Stem Cells *In Vitro* (Lab Cultured)

A. Differentiated Cells from Human <u>Embryonic Stem Cells</u>:

Embryo (H9 cell line) $\xrightarrow{\textit{GF (growth factors) + Cytokines}}$ *Neuron, skin, adrenal, blood cell precursors, liver, heart, pancreas, muscle, bone, kidney, gut, cartilage, epithelia, neural epithelia*

B. Differentiated Cells from Induced Human <u>Adult Stem Cells</u> (iPS Cells):

Bone Marrow $\xrightarrow{\textit{Transcription Factors OCT4, SOX2, KLF4, c-myc}}$ *Hepatocyte, myocyte, adipocyte, chondrocyte, red blood cell, white blood cell, neuron, cardiomyocyte,*

Brain $\xrightarrow{\textit{Transcription Factors OCT4, SOX2, KLF4, c-myc}}$ *Myocyte, astrocyte, neuron, oligodendrocyte*

Liver $\xrightarrow{\textit{Transcription Factors OCT4, SOX2, KLF4, c-myc}}$ *Red blood cell, white blood cell*

(Thomas C. Spelsberg Ph.D., 2013)

reprogramming. By removing or inactivating this protein in cells, almost 100% of the cells are induced/reprogrammed into iPS cells within a week.

To summarize, these iPS cells are more desirable for clinical use since:

• they do not involve embryos;

• they can be obtained with relative ease;

• there is no tissue rejection because these stem cells are derived from the host patient in need of new tissues/organs;

• when they are injected into the circulation of whole animals, the cells tend to localize into the tissues/organs for which the cells were directed by growth factors;

• they do not form teratomas (cancer);

• these cells appear to have the same regenerative powers as the embryonic stem cell; they can differentiate into all/most cell types;

• these cells have proven effective, relatively cheap to produce, and the most useful of all stem cells. The tissues regenerated by these iPS cells appear to be those of the patient and thus, avoiding rejection (see table 11.1 and figure 11.2).

F.   Issues and Applications of Stem Cells and Growth Factors/Cytokines in Regenerative Medicine

(1)   Growth Factors and Cytokines direct Stem Cells to Specific Cell Types

Exciting breakthroughs have also occurred with the identification of culture conditions containing specific protein growth factors and cytokines which can "direct" the stem cells to differentiate into specific cell types. These protein factors regulate embryonic (pluripotent), adult (multipotent) stem cells, and iPS cells, and direct them towards one cell type or another. These growth factor/cytokine treated stem cells are then "committed" and when they are injected into the animal models, they naturally hone in on the organ/tissue that they were designed to repair and generate the appropriate cell types of that organ.

Recently, a "rejuvenation factor", GDF-11 has been identified that can enhance the regeneration of brain, muscle, heart, liver, spinal cord, etc by stimulating adult stem cells. It is present in the blood of humans and mice but is much more abundant in young animals/humans. Wagers, Lee, and coworkers at Harvard in Boston have shown that this Growth Factor can essentially reverse aging in mice and even enhance the mental abilities including memory. Studies with humans are planned.

(2)   Embryonic (Totipotent/Pluripotent) Stem Cell (ESC): Ethical Issue and Uses

Table 11.4 summarizes the obstacles encountered when using stem cells in regeneration. As depicted in figure 11.1, mammalian embryonic stem cells are obtained from the inner cell mass of an early embryo called a blastocyst. These are cultured in the lab and shown to differentiate into many cell types. However, the use of stem cells from embryos causes ethical issues among the public, as well as biological problems.

Some proponents counter the ethical concerns with the following statements:

• embryonic stem cells can be obtained without destroying the embryo, and

• hundreds of thousands of unused fertilized embryos/blastocysts are destroyed each year world-wide anyway by in vitro fertilization clinics as unneeded, and discarded as waste.

To be more specific, the advantage of embryonic stem (ES) cells (pluripotent) is that they can theoretically differentiate into any cell type in the body.

Table 11.4

Issues and Possible Solutions to using Stem Cell Regeneration

Issue/Obstacle	Possible Solution
Immune rejection (graft – host disease)	• Use stem cells/tissues from same person (autograft or syngenesis (identical twin source).
	• Use immune suppressants for foreign regenerative cells/tissues.
Stem cell to desired tissue	• Use paracrine factors (growth factors/cytokines) to guide the differentiation to desired type of cell/tissue/organ in vitro (differentiation to alternate tissues can occur)
	• Allow partial differentiation to occur *in vivo* in patient or in another animal.
Wandering stem cells in wrong places (teratomes)	• Avoid embryonic stem (ES) cells that tend to form cancer like teratomas or localize in multiple places.
	• Can better use ES cells by allowing the stem cells to undergo partial differentiation before using, so cells will localize properly.

Note: Using genetically induced pluripotent stem cells (iPS) cells avoids
   many of the issues above.

(Thomas C. Spelsberg Ph.D., 2012)

The drawback is that they often form teratomas (i.e., cancer-like) blobs of cells throughout the body. Another drawback is the fact that ES cells from other donors can generate a negative immune response when injected into a patient as they are derived from another individual. Recently, Nelson and colleagues at the Mayo Clinic, devised a technique using genetic alterations to eliminate the preteratoma tendencies in embryonic stem cell populations. This should help alleviate a major problem in using any embryonic stem cell therapy. To be most effective, the ES cells need to be injected directly into the target tissues, or first be differentiated into partially committed adult stem cells in the laboratory with the help of growth factors/cytokines. In any case, the induced pluripotent stem cells are replacing embryonic stem cells in many studies.

(3)   Natural Adult (Multipotent) Stem Cell (ASC)

The natural adult stem cells derived directly from tissues/organs of a young adult, have proven useful in some therapies. The main limitation, so far, with many natural adult stem cell studies, is that they are not easy to isolate, difficult to obtain in large numbers, and they are limited as to what cell type/tissues they can produce (see figure 11.2 and table 11.4). These limitations are based on from which tissue/organ they were derived. However, the fact that these cells can be isolated from the same patient requiring a new organ/tissue and with improved efficiencies, is a positive aspect for eliminating the tissue/organ rejection.

(4)   Induced Pluripotential Adult Stem (iPS) Cell

As stated earlier, induced pluripotent stem (iPS) cells have many advantages over all other types of stem cells. These include: 1) the ability to use the cells from the same individual, 2) the ease to generate them, 3) their unlimited availability, 4) their minimal side effects to the host, and lastly, 5) such cells can be genetically manipulated before placing into the patient. Using the iPS approach, Dr. Terzic and colleagues at the Mayo Clinic and Cardio3 BioSciences in Belgium have recently developed cardiopoietic stem cells to reliably repair heart disease damage. This is a first for such a biotherapeutic cell line. These cells are genetically manipulated/differentiated to be more effective in heart repair. Many companies are now providing state of the art tools and services for the production of iPS cells for cell biology and clinical studies. For disease studies, there are companies that provide stem cell lines from humans with type 1 and type 2 diabetes, polyneuropathy, muscular dystrophy, glioblastoma, retinal diseases, Lou Gehrig's disease (ALS), and Parkinson's disease. In these stem cell projects, studies are ongoing to determine which genes can restore a diseased cell to a normal cell, using gene therapy technology. The companies also provide services to produce any stem (iPS) cell line from any tissue/animal of interest. They also provide a variety of growth factors and a variety of medias, to assist with targeted differentiation of these cells.

G.   A Summary of Important Scientific Developments

The scientific breakthroughs that have greatly facilitated the use for adult and iPS stem cells in regenerative medicine can be summarized as:

• When natural or induced adult stem cells, that have been isolated from specific tissues such as skin, are injected into whole animals, the cells have been shown to migrate, and localize to the targeted area. For example, partially differentiated, bone stem cells localize to the bone marrow, nerve stem cells localize to the brain, vascular stem cells localize to the heart and vessels, etc.

• Using specific antibodies recognizing a cell type specific protein, or sugar markers found on membranes of natural adult stem cells, scientists can now identify, and more efficiently isolate, the native adult tissue stem cells from the millions of mature/differentiated cells in adult tissues. Cell sorting machines efficiently isolate these native stem cells from a multitude of non-stem/differentiated cells.

- The most recent and major breakthrough in tissue regeneration occurred when induced pluripotent stem (iPS) cells were generated from differentiated adult cells by expressing several regulatory genes (coding for transcription factors) in fully differentiated adult skin fibroblasts and other cell types in culture. As mentioned above, and in table 11.1 and figure 11.2, these iPS cells:

1. can be redirected (differentiated) to almost any cell type;

2. can be taken from the diseased patients for study and possible gene replacement therapy;

3. have minimal negative side effects, e.g., no teratoma formation, nor immune rejection; and

4. can be genetically modified, e.g., gene therapy for a variety of diseases, before replacement in the patient.

5. Scientists are now investigating optimal conditions to encourage the proliferation of these iPS cells and to direct them to specific differentiated cell types. Using certain growth factors, cytokines (chemical messengers), and hormone/vitamins, the adult stem cells (and embryonic stem cells) can be differentiated into the desired cell type.

Chapter 12

Current Achievements in Regenerative Medicine

A. Introduction

This chapter outlines the current state of regenerative medicine, with a variety of organs and tissues, including its history and its successes. Regenerative medicine is in its infancy, but represents one of the most promising frontier fields of medicine. There have been not only some disappointments but also a lot of progress and much hope for the future of regenerative medicine. As discussed in Chapter 11, natural tissue regeneration naturally occurs to a limited extent in our bodies throughout life. The National Institutes of Health and the National Academy of Sciences have recognized regenerative medicine as the most promising component of modern medical practice. In the United States alone, there are 105,000 patients waiting for organ donations. All of these patients could be helped by organ regeneration.

Drs. Terzic and Nelson at the Mayo Clinic Center for Regenerative Medicine have deduced that the clinical usefulness of organ repair in humans relies on three general principles: natural rejuvenation by native adult stem cells, the long-standing transplant of organs/tissues, and regeneration of new tissues using stem cells. The following describes some of the advancements in regenerative medicine in a multitude of tissues and diseases that have been achieved. This chapter is divided according to the tissues and organs (in alphabetical order) so the reader can focus on specific areas of interest. For further reading on this topic, see the "References for Further Reading" section for this chapter at the end of this book. The author also recommends that the reader survey the internet for further information on this rapidly developing area of tissue regeneration. The studies reported in this chapter were current as of 2013.

B. Blood Cell Cancers

Research in regenerative medicine in blood cell cancers is a very active and ongoing endeavor in many medical centers. Blood cell cancers and the resulting radiation treatments require the rapid regeneration of these cells, much faster than the natural regeneration which normally occurs in our bone marrow to replace the eliminated cancer cells. The natural regeneration involves the differentiation of the bone marrow adult stem cells into many cell types: normal lymphocytes (white blood cells), myeloid, or lymphoid cells. Early trials involved the transplantation of bone marrow cells, which contain adult stem cells, into the same or another radiation treated individual with leukemia or non-malignant diseases such as aplastic anemia, sickle cell anemia, etc. However, the incidence of immune rejection using different donor cells was high and caused negative side effects.

The ability to generate adult induced pluripotent stem (iPS) cells from the skin, bone marrow, and other tissue sources from the same patient is now preferred, because the new cells would be recognized as one's own cells and eliminates tissue rejection. The iPS cells are generated, as described in the previous chapter, and allowed to proliferate into large numbers followed by partial differentiation into blood and bone marrow adult stem cells. The patient first receives massive radiation to eliminate all the cancerous and normal white blood cells. These cells are replaced with the patient's previously generated, normal, bone marrow (iPS) stem cells to replenish the patient's white blood cell population. These cells rapidly multiply to produce millions to billions of blood cells of all types in a short period of time. Current and future studies are also using iPS cells generated from the same patient's blood cells to regenerate solid tissues destroyed by cancer or those that had to be surgically removed. The immune compatibility issue with these iPS cells, of course, is avoided which is critical for success in all these replacements. This aspect is further discussed below.

C. Brain and Neurological Disorders: Parkinson's, Multiple Sclerosis, Alzheimer's, Huntington's, Lou Gehrig's Disease, Strokes

(1) Overview

Many neurological diseases are now being investigated for possible therapy for brain tissue and nerve regeneration. It is generally agreed that the more scientists understand the causes and development of these diseases, the greater chance of applying the best regenerative approach, especially if gene therapy on the stem cells is required. The adult brain is known to contain residual stem cells that are used for potential repair when brain tissue is damaged. The challenge is to remove scar tissue that often blocks regeneration. This is followed by triggering the local stem cells, or adding adult iPS cells developed from the same patient, which are directed to differentiate into mature brain neurons, without having unwanted cell types. This is achieved by use of appropriate growth factors (paracrine factors). Japanese scientists have regenerated mouse pituitary glands from stem cells using such factors. These could be used to replace diseased pituitaries, such as pituitary tumors. Studies in animals with brain damage have shown promise with injected adult and embryonic stem cells. Injection of these stem cells, which were already targeted to be neurons by growth factors, resulted in the repair of the neural damage.

Similar to the investigations in blood diseases, patients with neurological brain damage are now being treated with their own induced adult stem (iPS) cells. Recently, Swedish scientists have reprogrammed human embryonic and infant fibroblast cells, which were de-differentiated into iPS cells, to differentiate into neuro-transmitting brain neurons. These cells were shown to produce dopamine, raising hopes of curing Parkinson's disease. Blood cells are now being isolated, transformed to iPS (stem) cells, and the population expanded in the laboratory. These cells are either partially differentiated (targeted) into neurons and astrocyte cells in the lab, or injected into the brain of patients where they naturally differentiate into brain cells using endogenous growth factors to replace the damaged brain cells. After injection into the brain, these fresh, renewable cells will hopefully be able to alleviate many of the cognitive defects in humans, as they do in animals. Whether these cells can re-establish normal/complete circuitry and brain function remains to be determined. A recent report by Drs. Lancaster and Knoblich in Austria used human brain stem cells to regenerate small brain tissues with the natural brain lattice structures. This is a major breakthrough in brain repair.

Another goal of neurological research is to identify and replace defective genes in brain cells. Scientists are using animal models with human-like neurological diseases, isolating the host's own defective cells, transforming them into iPS cells, and growing these in culture. Any gene defects in these stem cells are then corrected by gene therapy or gene manipulation. Once corrected, the cells are re-injected into the brain of the diseased animals, eliminating most of the disease symptoms. In the future, these technologies could be useful in the future to treat Parkinson's, Huntington's, and Alzheimer's diseases. Using the iPS cells from the same patient that was targeted for brain cells, the regenerated brain would now contain new, genetically corrected, healthy, immune acceptable, neurons to help alleviate the disease.

Another novel area related to brain regeneration originated with the discovery of brain factors which, when injected into the brain, activate the formation of neuronal connections and improve brain cell activity. Some of these studies are being performed by Dr. Hench and colleagues at Boston Children's Hospital, Dr. Stritmatter and colleagues at Yale Medical Center, Dr. Wang and colleagues at Cambridge, and Dr. Davidson and colleagues at the University of Wisconsin-Madison. These activating factors, that increase brain neural connections, brain cell activity, and improve brain function, have been measured to be at the highest levels in newborns and during early childhood. Unfortunately, these levels begin to reduce as we age. Increasing these newly discovered factors in the elderly could one day allow the rejuvenation of learning, memory, and cognitive skills, using the patient's own cells. Dr. Davidson stated "Someday we will take responsibility for shaping our own brains." However, Dr. Pascual-Leone at Harvard has warned that "A system capable of flexible reorganization harbors the risk of unwanted change."

(2)   Advances with Specific Neurologic Diseases

Scientists, also using the induced pluripotential cell (iPS cell) approach described above, have recently redirected skin fibroblast cells into neurons with various specific functions. At the University of Wisconsin-Madison, scientists were able to generate motor neurons using this approach for use as a model to perform research into diseases that cause paralyses, including muscular dystrophy. Using both embryonic and induced pluripotent stem cells from humans, they generated human GABA neurons from these cells and injected them into the brains of mice with Huntington-like disease. The cells integrated into the brain, re-established the broken communication, restored motor function, and alleviated some of the Huntington-like symptoms. Imagine, a rodent with human brain cells. In other studies, neurons and astrocytes that were derived from skin cells of diseased patients, e.g., those with spinal muscular atrophy and Lou Gehrig's disease, displayed the same disease characteristics in culture, indicating that the defects in these diseases reside in each of the brain cells of the patient. Such cells are serving as unique models for laboratory research which involves the genetic manipulation of the cells to correct the genetic disease before reinjection into the animal.

Dr. Windebank and colleagues at the Mayo Clinic are using mesenchymal stem cells (hMSC) derived from a patient's fat cells to generate neurons. They hope to replace dead or dying brain/nerve cells with functional reconnecting neurons in patients with Alzheimer's disease, Parkinson's disease, multiple sclerosis (MS), and Lou Gehrig's disease. Scientists at Case Western Reserve University reported that they reduced the autoimmune response in multiple sclerosis (MS) and reversed the demyelination of nerves in a mouse MS model using human mesenchymal stem cells (hMSC). It appears that the normal hMSCs secrete a growth factor that assists in reversing the MS symptoms.

Studies are also ongoing in animal models with demyelinating diseases such as Parkinson's with the goal that injected "regenerated cells" (oligodendrocytes) will produce myelin to recoat the new neurons. Scientists at the Universities of California and Michigan were able to regenerate nerve and brain tissue in lab animals that have received radiation to create Parkinson's disease-like symptoms. The disease symptoms were markedly reduced after healthy stem cells were injected into the brain. The implanted stem cells in these animals differentiated into brain cells, replacing the dead cells, and reconnected with other brain cells. These animals are also serving as a model for humans who have lost brain tissue after receiving radiation to treat brain tumors. A similar therapy could be used in cancer patients whose brains are damaged by chemotherapy or surgery. Scientists in South Korea have recently transformed rat skin cells into neurons via the iPS approach. The cells were re-injected into rats with a Huntington-like disease. The rats displayed a restoration of motor functions. Similar improvements were achieved in rats with Parkinson-like disease. Scientists at the University of Michigan had similar positive responses after applying these same techniques to humans with Lou Gehrig's disease.

D.   Cardiovascular (Heart) Disease

While adult fish, amphibians, and mammalian embryos can rapidly regenerate new heart cells to repair large areas of damaged hearts, adult humans can only do so at a modest rate. Interestingly, human embryo and infants can more actively repair their hearts, even after extensive damage or incomplete development. This repair is due to the presence of an abundance of active stem cells in the newborn heart and blood. However, several months after birth, this natural heart repair in humans begins to decrease. Also, the hearts of pregnant or recent mothers have been shown to have enhanced ability to repair heart tissue. This was speculated to be due to the infant's adult heart stem cells circulating in her blood. These pre- and early postnatal heart stem cells have now been found in the mother's blood. A challenge for heart repair research and, ultimately, therapy in animal models is that any new regenerated heart cells/tissues require the cells to beat at the normal contraction frequency as do the native heart cells beat. This contraction frequency has ruled out the use of animal cells in human repair, because many of those heart cells are naturally programmed to beat at a faster rate than humans (greater than 100 beats per minute). Animal cells continue to maintain those rates even after cell culturing and transplantation. One wonders what mechanism in the cells controls this contraction rate.

Over one's lifetime, it is estimated that about one half of a human heart undergoes natural replacement or repair by endogenous adult heart stem cells. About 1% of the heart's 4–5 billion cells are replaced each year. The more of these repair capabilities, the better, as this ability would certainly enhance the survival of any species. However, these natural adult heart stem cells cannot replace the 1 billion cells lost in a typical heart attack as rapidly as needed, so additional targeted stem cells need to be added. Scientists are gaining expertise in isolating the rare natural heart stem cells from human heart biopsies. The number of these cells are expanded in cell culture in the lab and replaced into the same person's heart. A recent study by Dr. Riley, now at the Oxford University, reported the discovery of natural adult heart stem cells from the internal lining of the heart of lab animals were able to replace damaged heart cells.

Studies in humans with adult stem cells, however, have yet to show such success. This is due to the overall reduced number of adult stem cells and due to the slow rates of growth of the adult stem cardiomyocytes. There is evidence for an increase in heart growth factors in the blood following heart damage and repair. Interestingly, a natural heart growth factor (thymosin β-4) has been found to help heart regeneration, and encourage adult stem cells and iPS cells to differentiate into cardiomyocytes. Injecting this factor into animals with heart damage enhances the rate of natural endogenous repair even without the addition of stem cells.

Recent major advances in regenerative cardiology have been achieved in animal models. In one report, partially differentiated adult animal stem cells that were injected directly into the heart of animals with cardiac disease without any genetic manipulation or lab culture treatments, differentiated into heart cells (myocytes and fibroblasts). Major heart repair was then observed within 9 days. Dr. Zeiher at the Goethe University, Frankfurt, Germany, and colleagues, are using iPS bone marrow derived stem cells to treat cardiac disease in animals. A research team at the Gladstone Institute has inserted three heart specific growth promoting genes into heart cells to more rapidly direct animal adult cardiac stem cells to differentiate and replace damaged or dead heart cells. They demonstrated enhanced heart repair in rodents by transfecting these three heart specific genes in a vector construct directly into the diseased heart regions. These genes were incorporated into the native adult heart stem cell's chromosomes to activate repair. Similarly, scientists at San Diego State University performed gene therapy on animal heart stem cells to elongate their telomere domains of the chromosomes. This procedure also markedly activated the repair of the animal hearts.

Early studies (2008— 2010) with heart regeneration in humans used embryonic stem cells. However, as discussed in the previous chapter, ethical and medical concerns now support the use of the newly developed induced pluripotent stem (iPS) cells. The iPS cells, derived from patients' blood or skin cells, are manipulated to express tissue specific transcription factors and growth factors which cause them to differentiate into various adult heart cells including myofibroblasts and cardiomyocytes. Scientists in Israel have transformed human skin cells into iPS cells and differentiated them into normal beating heart muscle cells which resemble a new born infant's heart cells. Other studies have injected genetically altered myoblasts from the patient's own heart, using the iPS cell approach, to repair the damaged hearts, all with favorable outcomes.

Most intriguing are the recent reports that the replacement of new heart cells are not necessary to regenerate new tissue. Marban and coworkers at the Cedar-Sinai Heart Institute in Los Angeles found that it is the exosomes (tiny lipid bound vesicles secreted by the stem cells and carrying DNA, RNA, and Protein) that are involved in the heart repair. Thus it is not the direct involvement of the heart stem cells, but rather their exosomes that induce the regeneration.

Recent studies by Drs. Terzic, Belfar, and Nelson, with co-workers at the Mayo Clinic and Cardio3 Biosciences in Belgium, developed iPS cells from bone marrow cells of 45 patients from Belgium, Serbia, and Switzerland. These cells were stimulated with specific growth factors to partially commit them into cardiopoietic (heart) cells. The cells were then injected directly into the hearts of the same respective patients, resulting in a major repair of the damaged hearts. Increased blood flow and reduced heart volume were reported in all patients. Companies associated with these Mayo Clinic studies are Cardio3 BioSciences of Belgium, Mesoblasts of Australia, and Baxter of Deerfield, IL, as well as the European commission. Using adult mesenchymal stem cell and adult endothelial stem cell therapies in patients, several phase 3 clinical trials have been implemented by this collaborative team to regenerate cardiac tissue in patients with congestive heart failure, myocardial infarction, and myocardial ischemia. One phase 3 trial, called Chart-2, aims to recruit 240 patients in the United States with chronic heart failure. Overall, the stem cell heart patients treated with stem cell therapy display a 42% decrease in scar tissue and a 13 gram average increase in new heart tissue. World-wide, there are currently 12 or more other commercial companies that are currently involved in heart regeneration trials.

E.   Connective Tissue/Cartilage Repair and Related Diseases (Nose, Ear, Lips, Spinal Disc)

Lab directed tissue regeneration is now being achieved in animals and humans in connective tissue/cartilage repair. The regenerated connective tissues include vertebral discs, limb joints, nose, ear, lip replacements, etc. To achieve this, scientists are growing the patient's own chondrocytes (to avoid any immune rejection) on biodegradable molds mimicking the structures of vertebral discs, ears, or nose, or lips. Scientists are also using cartilage/connective tissue stem cells isolated from the bone marrow of the same patient, and partially differentiating them with specific growth factors to enhance cartilage formation.

Joints: There are 27 million Americans afflicted with osteoarthritis with many requiring joint repair. Free-floating stem cells have been injected into damaged or missing areas of the meniscus in the knee. The cells repaired the torn meniscus. New studies have identified the growth factors that specifically guide stem cells towards chondrocytes to produce specific types of cartilage. Examples are TGF-β, fibroblast growth factor (FGF), and Vimentin. Dr. Pee at West Virginia University and Drs. Li and Handorf at the University of Wisconsin-Madison have reported techniques and factors which can direct stem cells towards chondrocytes producing hyaline cartilage for joints. Dr. Marini and colleagues at the National Institutes of Health and Dr. Forlino at the University of Pavia, Italy, have identified a factor (kartogenin), that activates cartilage genes and helps direct chondrocytes to form new cartilage tissue. Using these factors, the scientists are growing cartilage on biodegradable molds to create discs in the lab to be inserted into joints and between vertebrae in animals. Human trials should not be far behind. The Center for Regenerative Medicine in Miami, FL, is already treating osteoarthritis patients with stem cells via direct joint injections with marked success.

Ears, Nose, etc.: The patient's adult stem cells have already been used to produce chondrocytes and epidermal cells which, in turn, had been cultured on biodegradable scaffolding made of collagen which match any structure: ear, nose, lips, etc. The latter repair is needed by accident and burn victims. When the ear or nose scaffolding is completely covered with the newly grown connective tissue with added skin, they are then attached to the patient. Circulatory vessels and nerves then naturally grow into these appendages.

Vertebral Discs: Scientists are using one's own living human vertebral disc chondrocytes to populate artificial collagen scaffolding which has been molded into spinal disc form. These regenerated discs are then inserted into the spinal column of model animals and shown to function as well as the original discs, eliminating the pain and regaining functions. The regenerated discs even integrated with local tissue similar to the native disc tissues. In related studies, scientists at the University of Bristol (U.K.) have obtained bone marrow stem cells as well as differentiated (transformed iPS cells) skin stem cells from animals, and grew them in culture in a biodegradable matrix that was molded in the shape of meniscal vertebral (disc) cushions. After growing over the scaffold, the cells were differentiated into cartilage cells using selected growth factors and cytokines, the discs then were inserted between the animal's vertebrae. These discs performed as normal vertebral discs. Currently, animals are mostly being tested, but in the future, humans with degenerative disc disease, torn meniscus, and osteoarthritis will surely be repaired by these approaches.

F.   Diabetes

Replacing whole organs is a more complex process since it involves the generation of multiple cell types, blood vessels, nerve fibers, etc. As described above for heart repair, studies in animals using embryonic stem cells to achieve pancreatic regeneration are also encouraging. Scientists have been able to differentiate embryonic stem cells into pancreatic beta (β) cells that secrete insulin. These are the cells that synthesize and secrete insulin, which will hopefully direct the appropriate utilization of glucose in the body. These "β" cells are either destroyed (type 1 diabetes) or lose the ability to produce and secrete insulin as in some cases of type 2 diabetes. The challenge is simpler with type 1 and in some type 2 diabetes cases, as opposed to other cases of type 2 diabetes, since these diseases involve replacing only one cell type, the pancreatic β cells. Scientists at the Gladstone Institute have recently reported the transitioning of iPS induced skin cells into stem cells.   These cells then differentiated into β cells which then restored insulin production in animals.

It was of concern that the injection of regenerated β cells from embryonic stem cells in animals often formed masses outside the pancreas. However, this did not appear to be an obstacle since these cells still functioned properly, producing insulin and responding to hormonal and metabolic feedback. In 2010, scientists manipulated human embryonic stem cells to develop into insulin producing pancreatic β cells – both from animal and human cells. When injected into diabetic animals, these cells formed cell masses outside the pancreas, but still produced insulin upon demand and thus eliminated the severity of the diabetes. Since embryonic stem cells often create teratoma formation (discussed in the previous chapter), the use of pancreatic stem cells generated by differentiated induced adult

257

stem (iPS) cells, has increased. Current investigations, such as those by Drs. Y. Ikeda, S. Russell, and coworkers at the Mayo Clinic, are achieving this feat using adult iPS cells generated from the diabetic patient's own bone marrow. This approach should avoid host rejection and abnormal growths (teratomas) at other locales which sometimes occurs with embryonic stem cells. The Mayo scientists are genetically altering the host pancreatic stem cells to produce the proper levels of insulin, which is required before injecting them into the patients.

Recently, scientists at the Universities of Massachusetts, Northwestern University, and the Mayo Clinic, used a type 1 diabetic patient's own iPS cells from his skin cells to regenerate the patient's pancreatic β cells. Some of these cell produced insulin when injected back into the animals and patients. These differentiated iPS cells behaved like normal pancreatic β cells with regard to physiologic regulations, resulting in all 8 patients showing improved disease recovery from diabetes. The future appears ready for the routine use of iPS cells from a type 1 diabetic patient's skin or blood cells to generate pancreatic β cells. These cells, when placed back into the same diabetic patient, should relieve or cure the disease without immune rejection.

G.   Immune Deficiency Disease

The immune system is comprised of over one hundred billion white blood cells of many cell types such as lymphocytes, macrophages, and others. These cells, which develop primarily in the bone marrow from bone marrow stem cells, are continuously replaced with new ones under the guidance of cytokines. Immune deficiency diseases occur by a variety of cellular defects that are corrected by replacing them with new iPS stem cells generated from non-defective stem cells, hopefully from the same patient's bone marrow or vascular system. These healthy stem cells originally were provided by a compatible donor, but currently, iPS (stem) cells from the same person are preferred. In cases of genetically inherited immune deficiency, the patients own diseased stem cells from the bone marrow have been isolated, cultured, repaired by single gene therapy, and re-injected into the same patient. This repair is discussed in Chapter 10 ("Gene Therapy").

Using technology of two fields of medicine, gene therapy and regenerative medicine, these gene therapy repairs of cells have been highly successful using this approach. The repaired patient's stem cells naturally differentiate into the full complement of now healthy white blood cells using this approach. The immune deficiency has been placed into remission within three months of the stem cell treatment, and the patients permanently cured. The immune deficiency diseases, including AIDS, remain a high priority target for this kind of therapy.

H.   Kidney/Liver/Thyroid Diseases: Regeneration of Whole Organs

Overview

Current research is ongoing to regenerate solid organs such as livers and kidneys, or at least the functioning cells of these organs. Organs under study are the heart and pancreas (discussed above), liver, kidney, brain, skin, the skeleton, and others in animal models. These tissues possess a natural ability to regenerate when partially damaged, even in adulthood. Of course, the younger the lab animal or human, the better the regeneration. Scientists have discovered that the surgical removal of scar tissue, or using host macrophages to eat away the scar tissue, markedly enhances the rate and extent of natural organ regeneration. An exciting new development has recently been reported. Using computer programming, scientists are creating 3D biodegradable scaffolds of cells mimicking those in animal and human organs with the hopes of growing new organs by allowing the stem cells to fill these scaffolds with differentiated cells for that organ. More accurate, native-like organs should be generated using this approach.

It is important to relate that the construction of an organ with all the normal cell types is not sufficient for a viable organ. The survival depends also on all the cells having access to oxygen and nutrients and the removal of wastes. Bischoff and coworkers at Harvard found that the addition of endothelial cells together with the stem cells directed for the organ's functions (e.g. liver, kidney, etc) causes the regeneration of tissues with normal vascular networks. Responding to growth factors from the stem cells, the endothelial cells form natural vasculature and connect with blood vessels of the host. Thus survival is assured.

Kidney: Scientists have used embryonic cells to regenerate a functional kidney in animal models. These cells/tissues grow into a cell mass that functions as a kidney, even though they do not resemble a kidney and do not have the normal blood vessels associated with the nephrons. Rat kidneys were also regenerated using connective tissue scaffold isolated from other kidneys.
These resembled a normal kidney. Dr. Ott and colleagues at Harvard University have regenerated human kidney cells onto a similar scaffold of a rat kidney. These were re-implanted into rats and have shown to function normally.

Liver: In the case of the liver, scientists are adding the patient's own adult stem (iPS) cells, generated from the bone marrow and skin cells, to surgically reduced or damaged livers to enhance this natural liver regeneration. Scientists at the University of Pittsburgh have injected liver stem cells into the livers of diseased mice to rejuvenate/replenish liver function. Interestingly, even though some of the liver cells grew in lymph nodes, they still functioned as liver cells and helped to replace the diseased liver functions. In another recent report, scientists at the

Massachusetts Institute of Technology, and in Japan, generated mouse livers using iPS stem cells from several cell types, including mouse fibroblasts, animal and human liver, skin, and endothelial cells. Even though the regenerated tissues did not resemble a natural liver in appearance, the re-implanted tissues of both animals and humans functioned similar to normal liver tissue after blood vessels grew back into the regenerated liver tissues. Obviously, regaining organ functions is far more important than regaining an organ appearance/structure.

Recently, University of Cambridge (UK) researchers created human liver adult stem cells from skin cells of the same individual using the iPS strategy. This is a major breakthrough as it had been difficult to encourage mature hepatocytes to regenerate the liver. Interestingly, scientists at Harvard University have recently developed a technique to generate a laboratory based liver organ in an animal model. This was achieved by stripping away of all cells from a liver, leaving only the scaffold/matrix. Using this matrix from one animal and the newly developed hepatocyte stem cells obtained from the target animal, normal functioning livers were grown in the lab for transplantation into the target animal with no immune rejection. This approach is being replaced by the 3D computer generated, cellular scaffolds of organs. As mentioned earlier, the addition of blood vessel (endothelial) cells to the regenerating tissue has been shown to markedly enhance the viability of the new tissue. These developments should allow tissue/organ regeneration of normal livers to replace diseased livers. Liver diseases are increasing in frequency and are often extremely lethal, leaving liver transplantation or regeneration as the only option.

Thyroid: Only a few studies have been reported as of 2013 for regenerating thyroid tissue. Dr. Costagliola and colleagues at the Free University of Brussels have recently grown functional thyroid gland tissues using genetically engineered embryonic stem cells.

Conclusions on Organ Regeneration: The regeneration of solid organs is more difficult and complex to achieve. Blood vessels and multiple cell types are involved. The fact that organ cells can function normally while not shaped as a normal organ and can function at other locales in the body is possible because the regulation of these cells occurs by hormones and growth factors circulating in the blood. The computer driven 3D scaffolds using iPS cells, capable of generating whole organs with the normal organ structure, represent the future of this field.

I.   Muscle Regeneration

As most of us know, muscle can naturally repair itself when small sections of the muscle are damaged. However, in cases where all or most of the muscle is damaged or removed, muscle regeneration is not possible. Recent studies by scientists have now identified that muscle tissue scaffolding (connective tissue on which muscle cells attach and organize) plays a big role in muscle regeneration. Dr. Rubin and colleagues at the University of Pittsburgh Medical Center are regenerating limb muscles in war veterans using animal muscle, and cartilage scaffolding. A trial using 80 patients is underway. Similar studies to repair rotator cuff damage and hernias are now being conducted. This extracellular matrix in cell organs/tissues seems to play a vital role in tissue repair, providing chemical signals and holding cells and tissues in the appropriate position.

J.   Peripheral Artery Disease (PAD)

Peripheral artery disease (PAD) involves the narrowing or blocking of the arteries of the lower extremities. Over 27 million Americans and Europeans have PAD. It occurs mostly in the elderly and diabetics. Normally in the young, arteriogenesis (artery repair) routinely occurs without any knowledge to the person. Diseases such as high cholesterol and diabetes encourage PAD, which develops by increased stress/pressure on the vessel cell walls. It is the lack of blood oxygen (hypoxia) that stimulates vessel re-growth (arteriogenesis). If severe, PAD often results in limb amputation, such as in the case of many diabetics. Bypass surgery, when applicable, is a current and effective therapy. Fortunately, tissue regeneration by stem cells is now being investigated for PAD patients. Several "proangiogenic" growth factors participate by enhancing the growth of endothelial progenitor stem cells residing in the bone marrow to generate new arteries. When arteries are blocked, and hypoxia occurs below the blockade, growth factors are secreted in response and trigger the enhancement of the proliferation and differentiation of the endothelial cells. These migrate downstream to sites of the blockage to initiate new arterial vessel growth.

Scientists are currently attempting to isolate, as well as generate, vessel endothelial progenitor cells from bone marrow, and multiply and differentiate these cells in culture using specific growth factors. Rafii, Nolan and coworkers at Weill Cornell Medical College have recently identified and cultured blood vessel stem cells that regenerate vessels when added into the circulation system. When these were re-introduced into the patient, a markedly enhanced arteriogenesis (regeneration of arteries) occurred at this site which bypassed the blocked site. A research team at the University of Helsinki has reported the isolation and growth of partially differentiated stem cells from bone marrow which can rapidly regenerate new blood vessels as endothelial cells. Early studies have demonstrated a marked repair of the arteries and improvement of muscle/limb functions when these cells were injected into animals and humans. Advances in the appropriate stem cell isolation and the addition of appropriate amounts of the cells into adult endothelial (blood vessel) cells should improve therapy. Reductions in immobility and limb amputations should occur in the immediate future. Interesting recent studies by Drs Coulomb and Murry et, al. at the University of Washington have identified a neurovascular guidance growth factor, SLiT3, which is secreted by adult stem cells and binds to the endothelial cells to guide them into blood vessels. Additional factors such as the vessel endothelial growth factor (VEGF) are needed as well.

K.   Retina

Currently, adult stem cells are successfully being used to create retinal cells in animals and humans. These cells have been injected into the back of the eyes of humans and animals and allowed to grow and differentiate. Some recovery of eye sight has been reported in animals and in humans. In 2010, scientists at the University of California-Irvine created an eight-layer, early stage retina in the laboratory using human embryonic stem cells. This regenerated retina had different cell types and appeared as normal retinal tissue at early stage development. Scientists at the University of Wisconsin-Madison have generated early retina structures using adult (iPS) cells derived from human blood, including light sensitive photoreceptor cells. In 2011, scientists at a small biotech firm in Massachusetts (Advanced Cell Technology) and at UCLA implanted 50,000 embryonic stem cells into the retinas of two blind women with macular degeneration, a progressive disease which leads to total blindness. Four months later, the retinas of these blind patients showed regeneration, and a year later partial eyesight was restored.

L.   Skeletal Regeneration

Natural stem cells from the bone constantly repair our skeleton throughout life to replace micro-fractures and weakened bone. Every 7–10 years our whole skeleton is naturally replaced via bone turnover and repair. Investigators are now able to differentiate bone marrow stromal cells into fat cells, bone cells (osteoblasts), and cartilage cells. Scientists are beginning to add enriched populations of adult stem cells from a patient's own bone marrow into selected (damaged) areas of the skeleton to enhance the repair of the skeleton. In England, scientists transformed human skin and fat cells into bone cells and created bone tissue in the lab. Scientists used these cells to create new bone for human transplants. Scientists in England have also regenerated auditory cells and cochlear bones which some day might restore hearing in deaf patients. Scientists at the Cincinnati Children's Hospital Medical Center have used fat tissue stem cells treated with the growth factor, BMP-2, to direct these cells to differentiate into bone forming cells (osteoblasts). They used these cells to generate facial bones and other skeletal bone for use in skeletal repair. Scientists are also targeting osteocytes with drugs to activate their initiation of bone formation.

M.   Spinal Cord and Peripheral Nerve Diseases and Injury Repair

Scientists have also been investigating the repair of spinal cord neurons and peripheral nerves. The latter have shown more promise, since nerve cells with severed axons often do not die, but, of course, do lose function. Current research involves the surgical removal of damaged tissue and creating a passage for natural peripheral nerve regeneration, and treatment with nerve growth factors to enhance the nerve regeneration. The spinal cord repair is more challenging since it involves the replacement or repair of the neurons, and the proper reconnections to target tissues and other nerves, as well as the insulation (covering) of this regenerated nerve with myelin sheath. Spinal cord repair may, in some instances, require the new challenge of having the large neurons in the cord regenerate their axons and reconnecting them to other neurons, as opposed to regenerating a whole new neuron. Using mice with severed spinal cords, stem cell scientists are having some success injecting newly differentiated neurons from stem cells to re-establish nerve connections. They are now including specific cell types, called "oligodendrocytes," to make myelin for nerve insulation (covering) which is required for proper nerve functions. A partial recovery of severed spinal cords has been reported within one week after the injury in these animal models.

More recently, Dr. Huhn at Stem Cells Inc., Newark, CA; and Dr. Curt, Zurich, Switzerland, reported the injection of human neural stem cells into human patients with spinal cord damage and paralyses has resulted in partial return of touching and muscle movement within weeks. Recent exciting studies by Dr. Franklin and co-workers, at the University of Cambridge Wellcome Trust – MRC Cambridge Stem Cell Institute, involved the injection of nose epithelial cells from dogs into the damaged spinal cords of handicapped dogs. The paralyzed hind legs became functional within a few months. Similar procedures have been used to regain hearing in human inner ears (Dr. Rivolta, et al, University of Sheffield).

N.   Skin and Bladder

Natural skin (epidermal) stem cells constantly replace and repair our skin from burns and injuries, as well as our urinary bladders, throughout our lives. For decades, scientists have been growing skin in the laboratory from individual burn victims. Obviously, these tissues/organs have an abundance of adult stem cells that produce the needed growth factors which have been maintained into adulthood for survival of the species. Starting with a patch of the patient's undamaged skin, and with the help of epidermal growth factors and cytokines to stimulate skin cell proliferation (growth), the skin is placed onto these burn victims with good success. One square inch of good skin from the individual burn victim can be grown in the laboratory to generate several square feet of new skin which is then used to replace severely damaged skin. Similarly, scientists have regenerated animal and human urinary bladders using host residual urinary bladder cells or bone marrow iPS cells.

O.   Windpipe (Trachea) and Esophagus

In Sweden, a patient with a cancerous windpipe (trachea) recently had his windpipe removed and replaced with an "artificial windpipe," made from his own stem cells that were grown on a man-made biodegradable plastic matrix. There was no rejection, because the cells were his own stem cells, which immediately began to divide and differentiate into adult epithelial/mesothelial cells. To give the windpipe a blood supply, the scientists stretched the stomach tissue with blood vessels up through the diaphragm to the new windpipe. These blood vessels and capillaries connected to the regenerated trachea. By 2013, over a dozen people have had tracheas successfully regenerated with their own stem cells implanted. The esophagus, like our stomach, skin, and blood, has constant cell turnover (replacement); therefore, it contains many adult stem cells which can regenerate. Recently, Dr. Jones and colleagues at the Hutchinson MRC Centre in Cambridge, UK, identified the natural adult stem cells involved in esophageal regeneration. These cells will surely be used for future esophageal and intestinal regeneration.

P.   The Potential to Regenerate Whole Limbs

Believe it or not, scientists have even been making advances in the regeneration of whole limbs in animals. Research into the natural limb regeneration in certain amphibians and fish has been ongoing for approximately 100 years. Over the past 13 years, the most rapid discoveries have occurred at the molecular level. Many lower-level evolutionary animals retain the capacity to regenerate parts of their bodies, including limbs, after birth. The more complex living animals (e.g., mammals, including humans), while often able to regenerate limbs *in utero*, lose the capacity to regenerate shortly after birth. For example, the severing of appendages of mammalian lab animal (rodent) embryos (*in utero*) results in regeneration of that appendage. This regenerative capacity ceases when the mammals are late stage fetuses or soon after birth.

Let us first address what is known about the ability of the adult amphibians and fish appendages to regenerate. The molecular and cellular mechanisms are currently being elucidated. As outlined in the flow diagram in figure 12.1, upon severing the appendage of a newt or amphibian, a cell mass ("cap") appears at the severed site consisting of mesenchymal stem cells. These natural adult stem cells resemble the man-made stem cells described earlier. Most of these adult stem cells ("blastema") are partially differentiated stem cells originating from skin (dermis). This differentiation affects nuclear reprogramming involving the activation of 4–6 regulatory genes, similar to the ones used to create iPS cells. Some scientists believe some of these stem cells arise from adult stem cells that are already present in the residual limb tissue. Other scientists feel these stem cells originate in the bone marrow/blood and migrate to the limb site.

Figure 12.1

The Steps in the Natural Regeneration of Amphibian Appendages (Arms/Legs)

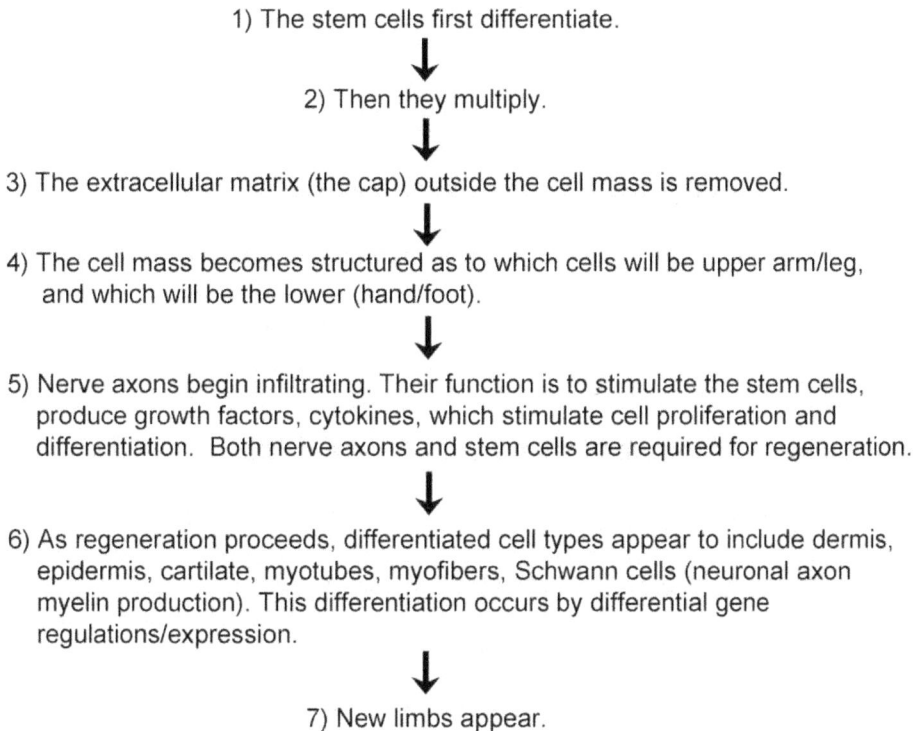

1) The stem cells first differentiate.

↓

2) Then they multiply.

↓

3) The extracellular matrix (the cap) outside the cell mass is removed.

↓

4) The cell mass becomes structured as to which cells will be upper arm/leg, and which will be the lower (hand/foot).

↓

5) Nerve axons begin infiltrating. Their function is to stimulate the stem cells, produce growth factors, cytokines, which stimulate cell proliferation and differentiation. Both nerve axons and stem cells are required for regeneration.

↓

6) As regeneration proceeds, differentiated cell types appear to include dermis, epidermis, cartilate, myotubes, myofibers, Schwann cells (neuronal axon myelin production). This differentiation occurs by differential gene regulations/expression.

↓

7) New limbs appear.

(Thomas C. Spelsberg Ph.D., 2012)

Animals that cannot regenerate limbs either do not form a blastema-mesenchymal stem cell group (cap) or fail to form a cap which regenerates partial appendages. In this case, cell de-differentiation does not occur and any endogenous stem cells fail to be "activated" to proliferate and differentiate. In short, all mammals and most animals obviously have, but do not express, the genes needed for limb regeneration. These genes, although present, and obviously expressed in embryos, are partially or wholly repressed in adult animals. Scientists have recently identified a gene in mice and humans, Lin 28a, that is expressed in embryonic and new born tissues, which initiates the limb regeneration. It is inactivated shortly after birth. Other studies by Alvarado and colleagues, at the Stowers Medical Institute, have identified a master regulator, a transcription factor, termed Fox-A, that appears to be essential to regenerate organs and limbs. This gene is conserved over evolution from flat worms to humans. Additional 20 lesser factors appear to be required for flat worms to regenerate themselves.

Interestingly, natural stem cells in animals that do regenerate limbs resemble iPS cells. In other words, they express the same pattern of genes as the inserted gene approach currently used in laboratories to achieve pluripotent stem cells. As described in Chapter 11, these gene patterns involve the same regulatory genes, e.g., c-myc, klf-4, sox-2, Oct-4, believed to create iPS cells. Each of these factors regulates a multitude of other genes coding for cytokines/growth factors. In other studies, scientists have used growth factor extracts from animal bladders to help regenerate adult human fingers after accidental loss. Obviously, such genes are repressed in the appendages of regeneration – deficient mammals. Maybe the re-activation of such genes at the sites of severed limb might allow the regeneration of limbs in mammals, including humans. Scientists are now attempting to use such techniques, including the important initiator growth factors such as fibroblast growth factor (FGF), to initiate limb growth. In rodents, scientists have sufficient knowledge to generate limbs. They can also generate at odd places on amphibians' backs, stomachs, etc.

Q.   Obstacles in using Animal Models

As exciting as all this discussion above sounds, there are obstacles to overcome, especially in translation from animal research to humans. Dr. Yamanaka and colleagues and Thomson and colleagues have discovered that the transcription factors used to reprogram mouse skin cells from embryonic stem cells had unexpected different functions than those found in human skin cells, sometimes with apparently opposite cell responses. These findings were unexpected. Similarly, as mentioned above, animal heart cells inherently display a much more rapid rate of heart beats compared to humans. These results obviously emphasize the need for direct human tissue/cell studies in the laboratory. Although most genes have identical functions in different animal species, a few display unique functions. In short, "what works for the goose may not be good for the gander" or "what works for rodents may not always work for humans, and vice versa."

Chapter 13

Epilogue: Assessing our Health and Hopes

In this book, we have described many aspects of the human body, the origins of the molecules of which we are made, the earliest life on Earth, the complexity of our body, the microbial (bacterial) world that lives in symbiosis with us, as well as advances of several important frontiers of medicine: gene therapy, individualized medicine, and regenerative medicine.

Humans (and all living entities) are comprised of the elements created in ancient, dead stars that existed before our solar system was created. The molecules that compose us are so small that there are trillions in each of the 10 trillion tiny cells in our bodies. In these terms, we are as complex as the cosmos. In our bodies, there are billions of chemical reactions ongoing in each of our cells every minute. Microbes, which represent the majority of life on Earth, are estimated to have co-existed on and inside our bodies and in all multicellular animals, beginning with our multicellular ancestors hundreds of millions of years ago. They now out-number our own cells 10 to 1. We now know that our symbiotic bacteria serve to protect us from "bad" (pathogenic) bacteria and viruses. They also help us digest food and regulate our health, immune system, metabolism, and even our mental state and disposition. As infants and children, they prepare us for life on this Earth, by helping to develop our immune system and prevent intestinal diseases (Crohns, irritable bowel, etc.). Considering all of the above, is it any wonder that curing human disease is difficult when one considers the complexities of the human body.

The genes (DNA) that carry the information to create each of us are invisible to the eye, and are so small that they all fit inside an 8 micron diameter (approximately 1/10,000 inch) cell nucleus. We now know that the protein coding genes, representing less than 2% of the total DNA in our chromosomes, are very similar to the genes of other mammals and animals. This fact is not surprising, since many genes code for proteins which carry out the basic functions of life. Most of the remaining 98% of the DNA (originally called junk DNA) is actually transcriptionally active and classified as RNA coding genes which are non-protein coding RNA (ncRNA). Thus, we may be dealing with 100,000 to over 300,000 genes in our genome. These are involved in the epigenetic regulation of the expression of the protein coding genes, as well as the RNA coding genes. In summation, the junk DNA codes for ncRNA, which included microRNAs, long non-coding RNAs (LNCs), and jumping genes (transposons). Along with other epigenetic regulatory genes, these contribute to make humans different from each other. This same regulation occurs in all animals, including mammals and many other types of living organisms.

It appears that defects in this "junk" (non-protein-coding) DNA may also be involved in causing many human diseases. Thus, the cure of many inherited human diseases will surely involve manipulation of the "junk" DNA genes. The complexities of the human body and the genes that control it are challenging to research investigators and have represented major obstacles in the past century contributing to the slowing of the progress in the cure of human diseases.

Considering these obstacles, progress in medical research is still being made at remarkable speeds. The assessment of disease predisposition, regenerative medicine, individualized medicine, and gene therapy represent the bright futures of medicine. The repair of damaged tissues, once a patch up job for surgeons, will, in the future, involve the use of natural tissue regeneration.

Advances in stem cell biology are allowing scientists to regenerate our own tissues in the lab and in our bodies. Thus, no immune rejections occur. The regeneration of aging or diseased tissues and organs will alleviate and cure many diseases, and extend our lifetimes significantly. The elucidation that each of us has some genetic uniqueness, as individuals, will enhance the accurate medical diagnoses and estimates of disease predisposition for all of us. This field of individualized medicine represents a promising diagnostic and therapeutic advance in medicine. It should provide more accurate and effective therapies for all people with afflictions. Finally, gene therapy should eventually provide cures for inherited, devastating, single gene diseases, and could even eliminate these diseases in future family members. These advances in medicine are progressing rapidly. They will enable humans, afflicted with major diseases, to live more normal, productive lives. Accompanying these advances, however, is the realization that Mother Nature's "survival of the species," would be partially eliminated, thereby increasing the frequency of the predispositions for disease in the human population.

The chapters described in this book, "Frontiers in Biology and Medicine," hopefully have generated excitement in the reader with the hope for the cures of many diseases, including the regeneration of failing tissues and organs. The author hopes that this book:

1) stimulates physicians, scientists, basic scientists, allied health care providers, and interested adults and young people;

2) encourages the youth to enter the fields of biology, medicine, and medical research;

3) encourages the lay science public to support medical research;

4) serves as a resource to educators and physicians and others interested in science;

5) instills an appreciation of life and its living organisms in all readers; and finally

6) gives an appreciation of the challenges that basic and physician scientists encounter when studying human diseases.

The medical advances described in this book are amazing in light of the uniqueness and complexity of the human body. A healthier and longer life expectancy is in store for the human species.

References for Further Reading

Many research articles, reviews, and news reports from the internet were also used as resources to provide as up to date information as possible. Author's names listed in the book, but not referenced, can be found on the internet under Google, Medline, Pubmed, library indices, etc.

Chapter 2: Cosmic Origins of Humans

Adams, Fred, 2002, *Origins of* Existence, New York, The Free Press

Emsley, John, 2001, *Nature's Building Blocks,* New York, Oxford University Press

Gaensier, Bryan, 2011, *Extreme Cosmos.* New York, Penguin Group

Galant, Roy, 1994, *National Geographic Picture Atlas of our Universe*, Washington, DC, National Geographic Society

Gibilisco, Stan, 2003, *Astronomy Demystified*, New York, McGraw-Hill

Hartman, William, and Ron Miller, 1991, *The History of the Earth*, New York, Workman Publishing Co

Hawking, Stephen, 1996, *The Illustrated Brief History of Time*, New York, Bantam Books

Sagan, Carl, 1980, *The Cosmos*, . New York, Random House, Inc.

Stwertka, Albert, 1996, *A Guide to the Elements,*. New York, Oxford University Press

Zeilik, Michael, 1994, *Astronomy: The Evolving Universe*, New York, John Wiley & Sons.

Chapter 3 - The Beginnings of Life

Carpenter, Jennifer, 2012, Multicellularity Driven by Bacteria. Science 337:510.

Liebes, Sidnwy et al, 1998, *A Walk Through Time.* New York, John Wiley & Sons

Reader, John, 1986, *The Rise of Life*, New York, Alfred A. Knopf, Inc.

Ronald, Pamela C. and Bruce Beutler, 2012, Science 330:1061-1063.

Siegfried, Donna Rae, 2001, *Biology for Dummies.* Wiley Publications, Inc.

Smith, Maynard and Eörs Szathmáry, 1999, *The Origins of Life.* New York, Oxford University Press

Southwood, Richard, 2003, *The Story of Life*. New York, Oxford University Press

Wharton, David, 2002, *Life at the Limits*, New York, Cambridge U. Press

Chapter 4 - The Micro-universe of the Human Body and the Cells that Compose It

Alberts, Bruce et al, 2007, Molecular Biology of the Cell, New York, Garland Science

Cooper, Geoffrey and Robert Hausman, 2009, *The Cell: A Molecular Approach, 4th Edition*. Washington, DC, ASM Press

Gartner, Leslie et al, 2011, *Cell Biology and Histology*, New York, Walter Kluwer, Lippincott, Williams & Wilkins

Gould, Stephen, 2001, *The Book of Life*. New York, W. W. Norton and Co.

Harold, Franklin, 2001, *The Way of the Cell*, New York, Oxford University Press

Knoll, Andrew, 2003, *Life on a Young Planet*. Princeton, NJ, Princeton University Press

Knowles, Richard V., 2010, *The Wonders of Genetics*, Amherst, New York, Promethius Books

Margulis, Lynn and Dorian Sagan, 1995, *What is Life?* New York, Simon and Schuster

Margulis, Lynn and Karlene Schwartz, 1988, *Five Kingdoms*. New York, W. H. Freeman and Co.

Wolpert, Lewis, 2009, *How We Live, How We Die*. New York, W. W. Norton and Co.

Chapter 5 - The Microbial World: The Symbiotic Social Life of Bacteria

Banfield, Jillian and mark Young, 2009, Variety: The Splice of Life - in Microbial Communities. *Science* 326, 1198-1199.

Ben-Barak, Idan, 1009, *The Invisible Kingdom*. New York, Basic Books

Betsy, Tom and Jim Keogh, 2005, *Microbiology Demystified*. New York, McGraw Hill, Inc.

Biddle, Wayne, 2009, *A Field Guide to Germs*, New York, Anchor Books

Bradley, Alexander S., 2009, Expanding the Limits of Life. *Scientific American*, Dec. 62-67.

Byrd, Jeffrey and Tabatha M. Powledge, 2006, *Microbiology: A Complete Idiots Guide*. New York, Alpha Publications (Penguin Group, USA, Inc.)

Dusenberg, David B., 1996, *Life at Small Scale (The Behavior of Microbes)*. New York, Scientific American Library and W.H. Freeman and Co.

Ewald, Paul W., 2000, *Plaque Time*, New York, Simon & Schuster, The Free Press

Gold, Thomas, 2001, *The Deep Hot Biosphere*. New York, Copernicus Books

Gross, Michael, 1998, *Life on the Edge*. New York, Plenum Press

Ingraham, John L., 2010, *March of the Microbes: Sighting the Unseen*. Cambridge, Belknap Press

Jacquot, Jeremy, 2009, Microbes. *Discover*, Sept. 12-13.

Knoll, Andrew H., 2003, Life on a Young Planet, Princeton University Press

MacZulak, Anne, 2011, *Allies and Enemies: How the World Depends on Bacteria*. Upper Saddle River, NJ, Pearson Education, Inc.

Madigan, Michael T. and Barry L. Marrs, 1997. Extremophiles. *Scientific American*, April, 82-87.

Margulis, Lynn and Dorian Sagan, 1986/1997, *Microcosmos*. Berkeley, University of California Press

Needham, Cynthia et al, 2000, *Intimate Strangers: Unseen Life on Earth*. Washington, DC, ASM Press

Taylor, Michael R., 1999, *Dark Life*. New York, Scribner & Sons

Tierno, Phillip, 2001, *The Secret Life of Germs*. New York, Atria Books

Waters, Tom, 1994, Life in a Rock. *Earth* 3(4):20-23.

Wharton, David A., 2002, *Life at the Limits*, New York, Cambridge University Press

Zelicoff, Ian, P. and Michael Bellomo, 2005, *Microbe*, New York, MJF Books.

Chapter 6 - The Human Microbiome: The Massive Bacterial World within Us

Ackerman, Jennifer, 2012, The Ultimate Social Network. *Scientific American*. June, 37-43.

Arrange, Terri et al, 2013, *Bugs, Bowels, and Behavior*. New York, Skyhorse Publications

Bray, R.S. 1996, *Armies of Pestilence: The Impact of Disease on History*, New York, Barnes & Noble

Costello, Elizabeth et al, 2009, Bacterial Community Variation in Human Body Habitats Across Space and Time. *Science* 326, 1694-1697.

DeSalle, Rob, 1999, *Epidemic: The World of Infections Diseases*. New York, The New Press

Dixon, Bernard, 1994, *Power Unseen*. New York, W. H. Freeman and Co.

Grice, Elizabeth et al, 2009, Topographical and Temporal Diversity of the Human Skin Microbiome. Science 324:1190-1192.

Johnson, Arthur, G., 2010, *Microbiology and Immunology*, Baltimore, Lippincott, Williams & Wilkins

Karlen, Arno, 1995, *Man and Microbes*, New York, Simon & Schuster

Lupski, J.R. and P. Stankiewicz, 2006, Genomic Disorders, Humana Press, Totowa, NJ

O'Rent, Wendy, 2009, Slime City. *Discover*, July/August, 60-65.

Qin, Junjie et al, 2010, A Human Gut Microbial Gene Catalogue established by Metagenomic Sequencing. *Nature* 464, 59-65.

Sachs, Jessica, 2007, *Good Germs, Bad Germs*. New York, Hill and Wang

Schugart, Jessica, 2014, Beyond the Microbiome: Mother lode: Superhero Sugars in Breast Milk make the Newborn Gut Safe for Beneficial Bacteria. Science News 11, 185:22-26.

Turnbaugh, Peter et al, 2009, A Core Gut Microbiome in Obese and Lean Twins. Nature 457:480.

Vijay-Kumar, M. et al, 2010, Metabolic Syndrome and Altered Gut Microbiota in Mice Lacking Toll-like Receptor 5. *Science*, 328, 228-231.

Yatsunenko, Tanya et al, 2012, Human Gut Microbiome viewed Across Age and Geography. *Nature* 486:222-227.

Zimmerman, Barry E. and David J. Zimmerman, 2003, *Killer Germs*, New York, Contemporary Books (McGraw-Hill)

Chapter 7 - The Human Genome: The World of Genes that Create and Regulate our Bodies

Alberts, Bruce, et al, 1997, *Essential Cell Biology*. New York, Garland Press

Avise, John C., 2010, *Inside the Human Genome*, New York, Oxford University Press

Burdon, Roy H., 1999, *Genes and the Environment*, Philadelphia, USA Taylor and Francis, Inc.

Calado, Rodrigo and Neal Young, 2012, Telomeres in Disease. *The Scientist* 5, 42-48.

Dudek, Ron W., 2010, *Genetics - Board Review Series*, New York, Walters Kluwer/Lippincott Williams & Wilkins

Hartl, Daniel L. and Elizabeth Jones, 2001, *Genetics*. London, Jones and Bartlett Publishing, Int.

Knowles, Richard V., 2010, *The Wonders of Genetics*. New York, Promethius Books

Lupski, James R. and Pawel Stankiewicz, 2006, *Genome Disorders*, Totowa, NJ., Humana Press

Pritchard, Jonathan K., 2010, How We are Evolving. *Sci. American*, October, pp. 41-47.

Qin, Junjie et al, 2010, A Human Gut Microbial Gene Catalogue established by Metagenomic Sequencing. *Nature* 464, 59-65.

Yatsunenko, Tanya et al, 2012, Human Gut Microbiome viewed Across Age and Geography. *Nature* 486:222-227.

Chapter 8 - Creating the Human Individual

Barbujani, Guido et al, 1997, An Appointment of Human DNA Diversity. *Proc. Natl. Acad. Sci.* 94:4516-4519

Baye, Tesfaye et al, 2009, Genomic and Geographic Distribution of Private SNPs and Pathways in Human Populations. *Personalized Medicine* 6:623-641.

Carey, Nessa, 2012, *The Epigenetics Revolution*. New York, Columbia U. Press

Lagos-Quantana, Mariana et al, 2001, Identification of Novel Genes Coding for Small Expressed RNAs. *Science* 294:853-858.

Lerner, Michael R. et al, 1980, Are snRNPs involved in Splicing, *Nature* 283:220-224.

Lewontin, Richard C., 1972, The Apportionment of Human Diversity. *Evol. Biol.* 6:381-398

MacArthur, Daniel G. et al, 2012, A Systemic Survey of Loss of Function Variants in Human Protein Coding Genes. *Science* 335:823-828.

Nelson, Matthew R. et al, 2012, An Abundance of Rare Functional Variants in 202 Drug Target Genes. *Science* 337:100-104.

Nussbaum, Roberg L. et al, 2007, *Genetics in Medicine*. Philadelphia, Saunders, Elsevier.

Olson, Steve, 2002, *Mapping Human History*, New York, Houghton Mifflin Co.

Pleasance, Erin D. et al, 2010, A SmallLung Cancer Genome with Complex Signatures of Tobacco Exposure. Nature 463:184-190.

Read, Andrew and Diane Donnai, 2011, *New Clinical Genetics*, Branbury, Scion Publishing, Ltd.

Sykes, Bryan (Ed), 1999, *The Human Inheritance*, Oxford, Oxford University Press

Tennessen, Jacob A., et al, 2012, Evolution and Functional Impact of Rare Coding Variations from Deep Sequencing of Human Exomes. *Science* 337:64-69.

Tobias, Edward S. et al, 2011, *Essential Medical Genetics*. West Sussex, Wiley-Blackwell Publishing

Visscher, Peter M. et al, 2012, Five Years of GWAS Discovery. *Am. J. Human Genetics* 90:7-24.

Wells, Spencer, 2006, *Deep Ancestry, Inside the Genographic Project*, Washington, DC, National Geographic Society

Wieben, Eric D. et al, 1983, UI Small Nuclear RNP Studied by in vitro Assembly. *J. Cell. Biol.* 96:1751-1755.

Chapter 9 - Foundations of Individualized/Personalized Medicine

Baye, Tesfaye et al, 2009, Genomic and Geographic Distribution of Private SNPs and Pathways in Human Populations. *Personalized Medicine* 6:623-641.

Collins, Francis S., 2010, *The Language of Life*, New York, Harper Collins Publishing

Knowles, Richard V., 2010, *The Wonders of Genetics*, Amherst, Promethius Books

McKenna, David H. and Claudio G. Brunstein, 2011, Umbilical Cord Blood: Current Status and Future Directions. *Vox Sang* 100:150-162.

Orlando, Guiseppe et al., 2011, Regenerative Medicine as Applied to Solid Organ Transplantation: Current Status and Future Challenges. *Transplant Int.* 24:223-232.

Passarge, Eberhardt, 2001, *Color Atlas of Genetics*, New York, Georg Thieme Verlag, Stuttgart, Germany

Robinson, Tara A., 2010, *Genetics for Dummies*, Hobokin, Wiley Publishing, Inc.

Russo, Francesco and M. Parola, 2011, Stem and Progenitor Cells in Liver Regeneration and Repair. *Cytotherapy* 13: 135-44.

Russo, Isabella et al, 2011, Effects of Neuroinflammation on the Regenerative Capacity of Brain Stem Cells. *J. Neurochem.* 116:947-956.

Wong, Sharon and Harold Bernstein, 2010, Cardiac Regeneration Using Human Embryonic Stem Cells: producing Cells for Future Therapy. *Reg. Med.* 5:763:775.

Wu, Yaojiong et al, 2010, Concise Review: Bone Marrow-Derived Stem/Progenitor Cells in Cutaneous Repair and Regeneration. *Stem Cells* 28, 905-915

Yin, Zi et all, 2010, Stem Cells for Tendon Tissue Engineering and Regeneration. *Expert Opinion on Biological Therapy* 10:689-700.

Yi, B. Alexander et al, 2010, Pregenerative Medicine: Developmental Paradigms in the Biology of Cardiovascular Regeneration. *J. Clin. Invest.* 120:20-28

Chapter 10 - Curing Genetic Diseases: Gene Therapy

Collins, Francis S., 2010, *The Language of Life*, New York, Harper-Collins Publishing

Cummings, Michael R., 2006, *Human Heredity*, Belmont, Thomson Brooks/Cole

Jorde, Lynn B. and John C. Carey, et al, 2000, *Medical Genetics*, Philadelphia, Mosby Publishing

Kaiser, Jocelyn, 2011, Gene Therapists Celebrate a Decade of Progress, *Science* 334, 29-30.

Knowles, Richard V, 2010, *The Wonder of Genetics*. Amherst, Promethius Books

Korf, Bruce, 2007, *Human Genetics and Genomics*, Malden, Blackwell Publishing

Nussbaum, Robert L. et al, 2007, *Thompson & Thompson Genetics in Medicine*. Philadelphia, Saunders, Elsevier

Robinsin, Tara R., 2010, *Genetics for Dummies*, Hoboken, Wiley Publishing

Russell, Steven J. et al, 2012, Oncolytic Virotherapy. *Nature Biotechnology* 30:658-670.

Chapter 11 - Regenerative Medicine: The Power of the Human Stem Cell

Buchheiser, Anja et al, 2009, Cord Blood for Tissue Regeneration, *J. (Prospectus) Cell Biochem.* 108:762-768.

Goldstein, Lawrence S.B. and Meg Schneider, 2010, *Stem Cells for Dummies*, Hoboken, Wiley Publications, Inc.

Panno, Joseph, 2010, *Stem Cell Research*, New York, Check Mark Books

Stocum, David L. and JoAnne Cameron, 2011, Looking Proximally and Distally: 100 Years of Limb Regeneration and Beyond. *Developmental Dynamics* 240:943-968.

Takahashi, Kagutochi et al, 2007, Induction of Pluripotent Stem Cells from Mouse Embryonic and Adult Fibroblast Cultures by Defined Factors. *Cell* 120:663-676.

Chapter 12 - Current Achievements in Regenerative Medicine

Baker, Monva, 2011, Neurons from Reprogrammed Cells. *Nature Methods*, 8:905-909.

Beil, Laura, 2011, Reviving a Tired Heart, *Science News* (Oct. 22):26-29.

Chin, Lynda et al, 2011, Nature Med 17, 297-303.

Flanagan, Nina, 2010, Stem Cell Studies go Forward Despite Some Opposition. *Clinical Research and Diagnostics.* (Jan 1):36-38.

Mehta, Rutika et al, 2011, Personalized Medicine: The Road Ahead. *Clnical Breast Cancer* 11:20-26

Neimark, Jill, 2009, The DNA Cure. *Discover*, 30:37-41.

Nelson, Timothy J. et al, 2008, Stem Cells: Biologics for Regeneration. *Clin. Pharmacol. & Therapeutics* 84:297-303

Nelson, Timothy J. et al, 2012, "Strategies for Therapeutic Repair: The R^3 Regenerative Medicine Paradigm. *Clinical Translation Science* 1(2):168-171.

Purnell, Beverly, 2011, The Complete Guide to Organ Repair, *Science* 322:1489-1510.

Scheiber, Joseph, 2011, How Can We Enable Drug Discovery Informatics for Personalized Health Care? *Expert Opinion on Drug Discovery* 6:219-224

Sneider, Erica B. et al, 2009, Regenerative Medicine in the Treatment of Peripheral Arterial Disease. *J. Cell. Biochem.* 108:753-761.

Terzic, Andre and Timothy J. Nelson, 2010, Regenerative Medicine: Advancing Health Care. *J. Am. College of Cardiol.* 55:2254-2257.

Tsonis, Panagiotis et al, 1996, *Limb Regeneration*, Cambridge, University of Cambridge Press

Yan, Qing, 2011, Toward the Integration of Personalized and Systems Medicine: Challenges, Opportunities, and Approaches. <u>Personalized Medicine</u> 8:1-4

Yandell, Kate, 2013, Organs on Demand, *The Scientist.* Sept. 38-45.

Zhang, Yong E. et al, 2011, Accelerated Recruitment of New Brain Development. *Plos. Biology*, 9:1-13.

Definitions

adeno-associated viruses: similar to adenoviruses, but able to infect a variety of dividing cell types with little immune rejection, but can only carry small pieces of DNA.

adenovirus: a non-enveloped virus containing double-stranded DNA and infecting mammals and birds, causing gastroenteritis and respiratory infections (colds, pneumonia). Efficient in infecting many cell types. Used here to carry large pieces of DNA into dividing cells and tissues for gene therapy.

adult stem cells (multipotent): stem cells in adult tissues that are able to differentiate several adult cell types.

algae: a class of protista, mostly single cell eukaryotes that live in water, most using photosynthesis as plants but others using chemical energy as animals.

Archaea: One of two subkingdoms (phyla) of bacteria. The other is eubacteria. Many of these live in extreme environments, and are called extremophiles. This subkingdom is thought to represent the first forms of life on Earth.

atoms: smallest particle of chemical elements that contains the chemical properties of that element; comprised of a nucleus of protons and neutrons surrounded by orbiting electrons.

bacterial (bio-) films: a community of microbes of different species attached to a surface and functioning in a symbiotic relationship; slimy appearance (e.g., dental plaque).

base/nucleotide: primary component of DNA or RNA containing a pyrimidine or purine base attached to a deoxyribose or ribose sugar respectively: one of the genetic triplet code of three bases.

chromosome: structures in the cell nucleus that contain the DNA (genes) and associated proteins. There are 46 chromosomes in most cells of the human body.

compound: substance formed by the chemical bonding of 2 or more different elements/atoms into molecules.

cosmos (universe): The universe, i.e., everything in the universe, including stars, planets, nebulae, galaxies, etc.

cyanobacteria (b-g algae): a phylum consisting of 2 groups of photosynthetic bacteria which use the sun to produce its food and energy, and use water to produce oxygen.

cytokines: see Growth Factors

diploid: cells or organisms containing two sets of chromosomes (one maternal set and one paternal set).

DNA (deoxyribonucleic acids): genetic material in the chromosomes of the cell nucleus containing hereditary genes comprised of deoxyribose sugars and the nitrogen containing base units.

DNA methylation: methylation of cytosine in/around gene domains that can restrict gene activity (gene expression); involved in the epigenetic regulation of gene expression.

dysbiosis: imbalances in the microbiome associated with human diseases and ailments.

elements: basic form of substances found on Earth that cannot be broken down.

embryonic stem cell (totipotent): totipotent or pluripotent stem cells in the embryo which can generate most (pluripotent), if not all (totipotent), cell types in the human body.

environment-induced mutations: DNA (gene) mutations and possibly epigenetic changes caused by environmental mutagens such as chemicals and ultraviolet light, and atomic radiation. Examples of such environmental mutagens are cigarette smoking, coal dust, and sunlight.

enzymes: a protein with the power to perform biochemical reactions at a high rate and specificity.

epigenetics: (meaning "above Genetics"); the study of factors and processes that influence (regulates) gene expression, but do not alter the genotype (DNA sequence); the regulation of gene expression (RNA and protein production) by mechanisms other than changes in the DNA; examples are: DNA modifications (methylation), histone and transcription factor modifications (acetylation, phosphorylation), and microRNA regulation of protein synthesis and mRNA stability; current analyses of epigenetic effects are measurements of mRNA and protein levels and enzyme activities.

epigenome: genes, mostly located in the junk DNA, that code for RNA, but not protein, and regulate the expression of other protein coding genes via epigenetics.

eukaryotes/eukarya: a kingdom of organisms composed of complex cells which contain a nucleus and true chromosomes represent plants, animals, insects, fungi, and protista: some scientists classify this category as a superkingdom.

exome: the combined exons of a genome; all domains in a genome that can code for RNA and/or protein.

exon: domains of a gene which are transcriptionally active and code for protein.

exosome (nuclear): a multi-enzyme complex involved in multiple RNA processing and degradation; involved in RNA turnover and half-life.

exosomes (extracellular): extracellular nano-vesicle originating from one cell and merging with another. These vesicles transfer lipids, DNA, RNA, and protein (in the form of regulatory RNAs, growth factors, and hormones) from one cell to another and often affect the biology of the neighboring cell.

extremophiles: any microbe (bacteria, fungi, protists) that inhabits extreme environments (e.g., heat, salt, acidity, pressure); they usually use chemical elements for energy and breathing.

galaxy: a huge cluster of stars (islands) numbering in the billions in the cosmos.

gene: hereditary unit in the genome (DNA in the chromosomes) that codes for functional proteins or RNAs.

gene delivery: the delivery of genes to cells/embryos using detergents, electrical fields, nano particles and viral particles.

genetic drift: periodic, spontaneous changes over time and generations in human (and animal) DNA; ultimately can cause changes in the appearance and physiology over many generations in isolated populations via environmental selection creating ethnic groups in humans, and thus, does play a major role in creating individuals by the inheritance of unique genes from parents; different animal species can evolve if the drift occurs over very long periods; since the mutations, environmental selection, and subsequent appearance of polymorphisms, due to genetic drift, occur at a very slow but relatively constant frequency; these polymorphisms can be applied to genetic tracking of human origins and world migrations.

genetic (parental) imprinting: expression of genes is determined by the parent who contributed them: one of the pair of genes (either one from the mother or one from the father) is expressed; the other is repressed.

genetic/genomic sequencing: the sequencing of the whole genomic DNA of an individual; this includes protein coding and RNA coding genes, as well as intron and regulatory domains.

genetics: branch of biology concerned with the creation of living species and their heredity.

genomics: field involving the study of the genomes of living creatures.

germ cell: sperm and egg cells of the human body containing only 23 chromosomes and function to join to create an embryo.

growth factors/cytokines (paracrine factors): proteins secreted by one cell to bind to membrane receptors of neighboring cells to regulate cell division and cell functions, including cell differentiation. Act as cell to cell communicators.

haploid: cells or organisms containing one set of chromosomes as found in germ cells, i.e., sperm and egg.

histone modification: side chain modification of histone proteins by acetylation, methylation, phosphorylation, and ubiquitination, which affects DNA condensation and gene expression; involved in epigenetic regulation of gene expression.

homo sapiens / sapiens: the modern species of today's humans: classified under the order "primates" and genus "homo."

horizontal gene transfer: transfer of genetic information from one species to another, as they live side by side.

human cells: basic living unit of human bodies (and all eukaryotes): a eukaryote cell type with protoplasm surrounded by a plasma membrane and containing a nucleus and mitochondria; there are approximately 200 types of human cells in the human body.

human genome: all the genes (genetic information) carried by a human cell.

identical twins (monozygotic twins): twins which arise from the division of the same fertilized egg to create two distinct embryos with identical sets of inherited genes.

individualized medicine: the new field of medicine regarding each individual as unique and requiring individualized diagnoses and treatments of diseases.

induced pluripotential stem cell: laboratory generated stem cells using 4 key regulatory genes inserted into mature differentiated (adult) cells which then cause the de-differentiation into a stem cell. Many cell types, e.g., the skin or bone marrow, can be used as a target for these 4 genes. These cells can then be differentiated into many cell types. They resemble embryonic stem cells. These cells allow regeneration of tissues in the same patients from whom the stem cells were generated, which eliminates rejection.

inflammatory cytokines: paracrine or hormonal proteins secreted mainly by macrophages involved in encouraging inflammation to combat diseases, pathogens, or abnormal tissues (cancer calcified tissues, such as heart valves); examples are interleukin 1, tumor necrosis factor, leukotrienes, fatty acids, and lipopolysaccharides; some of these are secreted by damaged tissues.

International Human Microbiome Consortium: a multinational organizational/ institutional consortium, collaborating to determine all the species of bacteria living in and on humans at various body locations.

intron: domains of a gene which are transcriptionally active (produce RNA) but do not code for protein in the pre-messenger RNA: RNA domains are removed from the pre-messenger RNA before protein production.

junk DNA: an erroneous term formerly applied to the non-functioning parts (90%) of the genome, excluding the protein coding genes. This domain is now known to contain pseudogenes, repetitive DNA, which includes transposons: approximately

75% of the DNA is transcriptionally active (RNA producing but not protein coding) whose genes code for small microRNAs, interfering RNAs, and long non-coding RNAs.

kingdom Animalia: represents all animals in the superkingdom; represents eukaryotes whose cells lack cell walls and undergo embryonic development of egg-blastula-gastrula-adult.

kingdom fungi: acellular eukaryotes that lack chlorophyll and function as parasites or symbionts.

kingdom Monera (prokaryotes): kingdom representing all the prokaryote bacteria, including the two phyla called eubacteria or archaebacteria; some scientists classify this category as a superkingdom.

kingdom Plantae: eukaryote organisms comprised of cellulose wall and chlorophyll; these organisms are autotrophs: organisms that synthesize their needed organic materials from inorganic sources using the sun or geothermal or chemical energy.

kingdom Protista: kingdom comprised of unicellular and multicellular eukaryote algae, protozoa, fungi, plants, and animals.

kingdom: highest level of taxonomic classification: includes prokaryotes (archaea and bacteria) and eukaryotes (plants, animals, insects, etc.).

lipids: small and large molecules comprised of chains of fatty acids, chains of carbon and oxygen with side groups sometimes attached; used in physical structures, signaling molecules, some enzyme activities, etc.

long non-coding RNAs (lncRNAs): long non-coding RNAs that regulate the protein synthesis of coding messenger RNA similar to microRNAs; a subclass of ncRNAs.

macromolecules: large, multicomponent organic molecule usually comprised of carbon atoms linked together [e.g., proteins, polysaccharides (sugars) and lipids (fats)].

meiosis: single whole nuclear (DNA) duplication in a precursor diploid germ cell followed by two successive nuclear divisions creating the haploid germ cells (sperm or egg) with half the normal set of 23 unpaired chromosomes.

microbes: microscopic organisms consisting of bacteria, viruses, or protists (e.g., prokaryote and eukaryote); many are pathogenic.

microbiome: population of microbes (viruses, bacteria, protists, spirochetes, and fungi) inhabiting in and on the human body.

microRNAs: subclass of ncRNAs; small non-coding RNAs each of which have different classes/functions; one primary function is to carry out epigenetic (gene) regulation by binding to mRNAs, preventing protein synthesis and encouraging the mRNA degradation; these small RNAs fine tune the mRNA levels and thus gene expression without altering the DNA (gene) sequence.

microRNAs, long non-coding RNAs, non-coding RNAs: see Chapter 8.

mitochondria: semi-autonomous self-reproducing cell organelle in eukaryotes that provide energy and oxidation for the cell. These organelles have properties similar to bacteria and may have evolved from them.

mitosis: the total chromosome duplication followed by a single division of a diploid (somatic) cell resulting in two identical cells each of which has the normal (diploid) number of 46 chromosomes; occurs in many adult cells/tissues in the human body throughout a lifetime.

molecules: the smallest units of a compound that maintains the chemical properties that compound; a group of atoms forming a stable unit, i.e., a compound that can be divided.

monogenic diseases: rare diseases caused by mutations/defects in one essential gene; inactivation of these genes cause debilitating diseases that are excellent candidates for cure by gene therapy.

natural adult stem cell (multipotent): stem cells naturally occurring in adult tissues that are able to differentiate into several specific adult cell types of that tissue or organ.

non-coding RNA (ncRNA): the term describing all the RNAs which do not code for proteins. These RNAs are transcribed from genes in the "junk DNA" and are involved in epigenetic regulation of the protein coding genes. Examples are the microRNAs and long non-coding RNAs: ribosomal and transfer RNAs are not included.

nova: a relatively small star that explodes within milliseconds, creating heavier atomic elements, and over a period of weeks or months becoming thousands of times brighter.

nucleic acids: see DNA and RNA in Chapter 3.

nucleofusion/nucleosynthesis: The combining of lighter-smaller atoms of elements into heavier, larger atoms to create new elements under extremes of temperatures and pressures - occurs in the centers of stars during their life and during their exploding deaths.

nucleus: an organelle in a eukaryote cell with 10% of the cell volume containing the cell's chromosomes with DNA (genetic information), as well as the DNA replication and gene expression machinery.

omics: the total amount of something (Greek): see table 7.6 for list and definitions of various omics.

ontogeny: the complete developmental process of an organism.

organic molecules: molecules produced by living organisms that are comprised of carbon, hydrogen, and sometimes oxygen, nitrogen, and phosphorus.

paracrine and cytokine factors (see growth factors): chemical signal molecules which act as cell-to-cell communicators between cells; can be a neurotransmitter or hormone. Involved in regulating cell differentiation and cell metabolism.

paracrine factors: see growth factors

pathogenic bacteria: also called "bad" bacteria or disease-causing bacteria.

pathogens: any disease causing parasite – bacterial, viral, fungal, or protozoa.

periodic table: a table listing the elements according to increasing atomic number, which is based on the numbers of protons in their nuclei - the arrangement correlates with their chemical and physical properties.

phylums: primary taxon (subgroup) of kingdoms.

polygenic diseases: all common genetic diseases (i.e., those not caused by virus or bacterial infections or single gene defect) that are predisposed/caused by several to several defective genes; these defects can be DNA base changes or epigenetic expression changes.

probiotics: substances (foods/yogurt or pills) containing bacterial populations beneficial for the digestive system that help maintain a healthy digestive system by combating pathogenic bacteria.

prokaryotes (bacteria): compose the kingdom of Monera, which do not contain a nucleus or true chromosomes; the other superkingdom is eukaryotes.

proteins: large molecules comprised of linear chains of amino acids. These chains fold to create specific structures, some as components in structures in the cell, some to carry out enzymatic (chemical) reactions.

quorum sensing: phenomenon in which a population of bacteria produces and responds to intercellular chemical signals whose concentration indicates the density and the species of the cellular population nearby; their genes often respond to these signals in order to relate symbiotically and coordinate their actions for mutual benefit of the community.

regenerative medicine: the medical field that uses stem cells to repair damaged or dead tissues or organs.

repeat sequences: nucleotide sequences that occur repeatedly in the chromosomal DNA (genome): up to 70% of the genome is represented as repetitious sequence families, much of which is created by retrotransposons.

retrotransposons: one kind of transposable elements which replicates itself via RNA intermediates to create extra copies of itself which reinserts elsewhere in the genome; they create repeat sequences; probably originating with viral infections eons ago.

retroviruses: viruses comprised of single-strand RNA animal viruses encoding a reverse transcriptase to produce DNA which then is inserted into host cell genome. Used to carry genes into non-dividing cells and tissues.

RNA (ribonucleic acid): single stranded nucleic acid and ribose sugar containing bases; has multiple functions such as gene expression and cellular structures.

single nucleotide polymorphisms (SNPs): changes of a single base nucleotide in the DNA found in the human genome.

somatic cell: cells of the body containing 46 chromosomes (diploid). See also germ cell.

somatic stem cell: same as natural adult stem cell above. One of mitotically active, undifferentiated (i.e., uncommitted) somatic "stem" cells in most adult tissues that can replenish several different cell types, allowing natural tissue regeneration (e.g., skin repair).

species: a taxonomic category consisting of closely related individuals which can interbreed to produce fertile offspring.

supernova: The explosion of a large star - (eight or more times the mass of our sun), that fuses under extreme conditions, the nuclei of lighter elements to create the heaviest of elements, i.e., iron and all those heavier than iron. This occurs in milliseconds to seconds. Temperatures in the billions of °F and pressures 100 billion times that of Earth's gravity create these heavier elements. Supernovae are extremely bright, brighter even than the whole galaxy comprised of 100-200 billion stars; the brightness lasts a few weeks.

symbiosis: kingdoms, phyla, and species living together in permanent or prolonged close association with mutual benefits for both species (e.g., bacterial plaques and biofilms).

telomeres: a specialized sequence structure found at the ends of eukaryote chromosomes; structure (domain) contains a small sequence that is repeated up to 60 times but is gradually reduced as cells divide; when shortened, the cells cease to divide and undergo apoptosis; immortal stem cells maintain their telomeres using telemerase enzyme or another unknown mechanism to repair/re-lengthen the telomeres.

transposable elements (transposons/jumping genes): class of DNA sequences that replicates itself with the new DNA copy moving from one chromosome domain to another or from chromosome to chromosome; there are several subclasses of this class, often creating repeat sequences and affecting gene expression by inserting its copy near a gene to regulate its transcription.

transposons: one of a kind transposable elements which are flanked by repeat sequences. Usually contain functional genes in the middle and often regulate genes neighboring the insertion site.

universe: see cosmos above.

<u>Index of Terms</u>

www.ingramcontent.com/pod-product-compliance
Lightning Source LLC
Chambersburg PA
CBHW051205200326
41519CB00025B/7009